from PROGRAM *to* PRACTICE

A Guide to the Physician Assistant Profession

American Academy of Physician Assistants
950 North Washington Street, Alexandria, VA 22314-1552

Phone 703/836-2272   Fax 703/684-1924
E-mail *aapa@aapa.org*   Web *www.aapa.org*

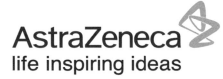

AstraZeneca
life inspiring ideas

Publication of this guide was made possible
by a grant from AstraZeneca

Cover photo: Andrea Holloway as a PA student. Andrea graduated from Howard University, Washington, D.C., in 2005.

Table of Contents

Section I

INTRODUCTION

Congratulations. You are about to complete your physician assistant education and begin the next phase of your life — as a practicing PA — joining the more than 55,000 professionals serving on health care teams throughout the world.

The American Academy of Physician Assistants has prepared *From Program to Practice: A Guide to the Physician Assistant Profession* to help you with the transition from being a student to becoming a practicing PA. A checklist is provided to highlight the key steps in the process and allow you to track your progress. It provides you with information about such things as certification, malpractice insurance, licensing, and employment.

You will want to personalize your checklist by making notes on it so that all the details will be contained in one place. The notes might include the following: the people you talked with about a specific topic and when the conversation took place; the phone numbers, e-mail addresses,
or Web site addresses you have used for references and to find information; and any other specifics that you need for follow-up and when you should do that.

However, the scope of this book is not limited to graduating students, as the information is relevant for any PA and will remain a reference tool for you in the future as you negotiate a salary increase, need a reference about medical staff bylaws, or consider accepting a job in a different practice. You might even want to refer back to the notes that you wrote on the checklist related to your license, certification, or employment.

Remember the checklist is a starting point and you will want to read through the related sections in the book for details on each point of the checklist.

Additional references on specific topics, such as the Guidelines for Ethical Conduct for the PA Profession or a list of state regulatory agencies, are provided in the back of the book, in the Tools and Resources section.

AAPA's Web site (*www.aapa.org*) is another source for a wealth of current information on topics related to PAs or the profession. You can also call AAPA's national office, 703/836-2272, and speak with the knowledgeable staff there about your questions.

GETTING STARTED: A CHECKLIST

ONCE YOU HAVE GRADUATED ...

☐ Create a professional file

☐ Create a résumé or curriculum vitae (CV)

☐ Request official transcripts from your program

☐ Consider repayment of student loans
 • AAPA's loan consolidation offer
 • Programs that assist with loan repayment based on qualifications, such as agreeing to work in a rural area for a specific period of time

☐ Sign up to take the PANCE and study for it

☐ Change AAPA student membership to AAPA fellow membership

_____

_____

_____

THE JOB SEARCH

☐ Review The PA Job Link and *AAPA News* for job notices

☐ Request an AAPA Salary profile for areas you are considering

☐ Create list of items you deem important and want to look for in a job (specific hours or days, salary, benefits, location) and rank them by importance prior to a job interview

_____

_____

_____

THE JOB INTERVIEW — WHAT TO LOOK FOR

☐ Check if employer pays for NCCPA certification/recertification, licensing fees, hospital medical staff fees, DEA registration fees, CME fees and travel, and professional association memberships (national, state chapter, specialty organization)

☐ Compensation (percentage of revenue, flat rate, profit-sharing)

☐ Personal/fringe benefits (health, dental, and life insurance; leave; disability)

☐ Malpractice insurance

☐ Schedule (hours and days work, on-call, flexibility, holidays)

☐ Locations where work

☐ Physician's expectations of what you will be doing

☐ Relocation and interview expenses reimbursed

☐ Timing of performance reviews

☐ Stipulations with contracts, such as restrictive covenant

_____

_____

_____

ACCEPTING A JOB

☐ Review contract and make sure it is what was agreed upon

☐ Compare with other job offers

_____

_____

_____

_____

_____

BEFORE STARTING TO PRACTICE ...

☐ State license (in most states, a new graduate license in available for a time period between graduation and receiving the results of PANCE)

☐ NCCPA certification

☐ Medicare PIN (provider identification number)

☐ Medicaid provider number (if required in your state)

☐ Provider number for private insurance companies accepted at your practice or authorization to bill under your supervising physician's provider number if the company does not give numbers to PAs

☐ Malpractice insurance

☐ DEA number (if prescribing controlled substances)

☐ State controlled substance number (required in some states)

☐ Delegation agreement or any other state-required agreements with your supervising physician

☐ Hospital privileges

☐ Copy of state statute and administrative rules that govern practice

_____

_____

_____

TO CONTINUE YOUR PROFESSIONAL GROWTH ...

☐ Keep your professional file up-to-date

☐ Read *The Journal of the AAPA* and *AAPA News* to keep up-to-date on the most current information related to the profession

☐ Track your CME on a calendar or in a file so it's easier to log the hours later

☐ Keep an expense record with receipts for all professional expenses (dues, equipment, etc.)

☐ Keep a procedure log

☐ Renew and maintain your license(s) and certifications

☐ Get involved with your national, state, and constituent organizations

_____

_____

_____

Section II

THE JOB SEARCH

While the stress of total immersion in clinical training may make the thought of job hunting seem laughable, the time to start planning an employment strategy is not when you cross the stage at graduation.

By the time you start clinical rotations, you should be thinking about what type of job you would like to have when you begin practicing as a PA. This does not mean that you should necessarily know the answer to the question (you may learn a lot about that during rotations), but you should start putting a strategy in place. Consider, for instance, that nearly one-third (31 percent) of respondents surveyed during AAPA's 2005 annual conference reported that they were hired by an organization where they spent time during their clinical rotations. That means contacts you make during rotations could prove to be very valuable later. It also means you may want to plan any discretionary rotations in a location or specialty of particular interest to you.

As you start rotations (or your second year of PA school, if your rotations are not all in year two), you may want to begin drafting a résumé, adding clinical experience as you move from one rotation to another. Early in the rotations, you might also want to take a look at the employment resources available on the AAPA's web site, *www.aapa.org/gandp/index.html* and *www.aapa.org/joblink/candidates.html*. Another valuable resource for PA job hunters is the AAPA publication Contacts and Contracts, available through the on-line AAPA Store at *www.aapa.org/aapastore/index.html*.

If you know the state in which you plan to practice, downloading and reading the PA practice act (link from *www.aapa.org/gandp/statelaw.html*) is an excellent way to prepare for job interviews and for practice.

Finally, remember the importance of personal contacts and networking. Communicate with people you know such as friends, relatives, business acquaintances, people at your rotation sites, and PA program alumni. Let them know you are looking for a job, and ask them to help you by letting you know if they hear of any opportunities. Most jobs are not found through employment ads or recruiters, but through word of mouth and personal connections.

THE PA JOB LINK
www.aapa.org/joblink

The PA Job Link is a comprehensive employment resource for PA students and PAs seeking a range of services, including job postings, salary profiles, interviewing tips, and contract templates to assist in negotiating an employment package. Accessible on the AAPA Web site 24 hours a day, 7 days a week, The PA Job Link brings the power of the Internet to your career search.

This is a one-stop site where you can search for employment opportunities, post résumés, and find links to related AAPA employment services. You can search for jobs by geographic location, specialty discipline, and key words. Best of all, it is completely FREE to PA candidates!

Here are some of the employment resources available to you at The PA Job Link.
- Manage your profile on one page. Your Career Page is easy to use and provides complete summary information – all in one place.
- Accurately track your current and past activity.
- View jobs or post résumés free of charge.
- Post a résumé — confidentially if you wish.
- Access hundreds of job listings locally, regionally, and nationally.

- View job listings 24 hours a day, 7 days a week — updated regularly.
- Send a cover letter with résumé when responding to a job posting.
- Receive e-mail notification of new job postings.
- Access personal assistance, toll-free, five days a week.

AAPA also provides you with the following essential tools:
- Cover letter templates and samples
- Interview preparation information
- Salary and benefits data
- Contract, liability, and business resources
- Many additional professional practice resources

The PA Job Link also offers personalized customer service assistance that is available Monday through Friday, 9:00 a.m. to 7:00 p.m. EST, at 888/884-8242; e-mail, *employers@healthecareers.com*.

The American Academy of Physician Assistants is member of the HEALTHeCAREERS Network, an intergrated network of prestigious association career programs, which includes the American College of Cardiology, American College of Allergy, Asthma and Immunology, and the Medical Group Management Association.

RÉSUMÉS & CVS

The résumé or curriculum vitae (CV), depending on which style you choose, is typically the first opportunity PAs have to make an impression on potential employers. A résumé is a condensed list, usually one or two pages, highlighting and summarizing previous and current jobs or other relevant experience. A CV is a longer, more detailed document designed to demonstrate expertise and authority that encompasses work history, education, credentials, and accomplishments, including articles published.

Should you use a CV or a résumé? It is most likely that, as a new PA graduate seeking a clinical position, you will be utilizing a résumé. CVs are used more in scientific and academic settings in which it is necessary to provide detailed information about activities like teaching, research, publications, and presentations. AAPA's *Contacts and Contracts* publication contains samples of well-written PA résumés and CVs.

Here are some helpful tips to follow when writing your résumé:

WRITING YOUR RÉSUMÉ

- Keep your résumé to one or two pages.
- Put your name, address, and phone number on the top of the page.
- Employment history should be in chronological order, beginning with the present.
- Include the dates of employment, job titles, and responsibilities in your employment history.
- Include relevant volunteer or community work. Avoid work that may be considered controversial.
- Summarize military in clear, civilian terms with no abbreviations. Write it so an individual with no military experience with be able to understand it.
- Include summer jobs as well as unpaid internships in a related field.
- Use a lot of key words — action words such as "mastered," "completed," "responsible," and "increased," and self-descriptive words such as "adaptable," "dynamic," "disciplined," "efficient," "productive," and "resourceful."
- Know exactly what you want and tailor your résumé toward that goal.
- Target your résumé for each potential employer.

APPEARANCE

- Use a font that is easy to read and avoid the use of unconventional fonts.
- Use a medium font size — typical font sizes are between 11 pt. and 12 pt.
- Use a good quality paper stock.
- Be sure there are no smudges, dots, or other flaws on the paper.
- Use only one side of the paper to print.
- Double check use of grammar and correct spelling.
- Do not use the subjective personal pronoun "I."

COVER LETTER

- A cover letter should always accompany a résumé.
- Cover letters should always be addressed to an individual, not "To Whom This May Concern" or "Hiring Manager." Contact the Human Resources Department of the potential employer to find out to whom the letter should be addressed.
- Do not rehash your résumé in your letter; it should be a complement to your résumé. Use it to highlight the aspects of your résumé that are relevant to the position and how you can contribute to the company.
- Use the first paragraph of the letter to grab the potential employer's attention and immediately address why you are a good fit for the position.
- If you have any gaps in your employment history, use the cover letter to provide an explanation.
- Double check correct use of grammar and spelling.
- Use the same paper stock as your résumé to print your cover letter, with a corresponding envelope, if mailing.

PREPARATION FOR THE INTERVIEW

The job interview is your chance to market yourself to an employer, to show them why you are the best candidate for the job. It's also your chance to get an understanding of the practice or organization, although you should research as much information as possible about the organization before the interview. You will impress your potential employer if you are knowledgeable about his or her business. You may begin the process by interviewing with a personnel officer or practice manager, but it's essential that at some time during the process you spend time with the person(s) who will be your supervising physician(s).

The interviewing process for some jobs may be made up of a series of interviews. For others, it may only consist of one or two. The questions you will be asked may be fairly straightforward, but you should be prepared for more probing questions. You should ask questions that will help you ascertain whether you will be comfortable with the work environment.

There are many resources on the AAAP Web site to help you prepare. For general Q&As about the profession, go to *www.aapa.org/geninfo1.html* or *www.aapa.org/members/pr/qa00.html*. For information about the physician-PA team, go to *www.aapa.org/gandp/issuebrief/pateamb.pdf*. The answers to many professional practice questions can be found on the Government and Professional Affairs page at *www.aapa.org/gandp/index.html*. There also will be information of interest to employers on The PA Job Link page at *www.aapa.org/joblink*. If the physician has not worked with a PA before, you may wish to take along some issue briefs about PA practice that are available at *www.aapa.org/gandp/pro-issues.html#ib*.

You should be knowledgeable about the laws and regulations governing PA practice in the state in which you hope to practice. You may want to take a copy of the state law with you to leave for the employer if they do not already have a copy. Links to all the state PA practice acts can be found at *www.aapa.org/gandp/statelaw.html*. You should also be prepared to provide a list of references, as well as copies of your relevant certificates (PA program, NCCPA). Before you interview, you should also go on-line and download or request a licensure application packet from the state in which you plan to practice. You will find this on the same site as the PA practice act. By reviewing the licensure application ahead of time, you will know what the process involves and whether the supervising physician has to submit paperwork.

As you research and interview for positions, look for a balance of quality of life, quality of practice (autonomy, philosophy), and level of compensation. Following an interview, you should send a thank-you letter to reaffirm your interest in the position and once again highlight your qualifications and the contributions you can make to the organization. You should also send a letter if the position no longer interests you so that the employer will not spend more energy on your behalf.

Contacts and Contracts: An Employment Guide for Physician Assistants, AAPA publication no. 180

TYPICAL QUESTIONS AN INTERVIEWER MAY ASK YOU

- What are some of your strengths? Weaknesses? Career goals?

- Why do you feel you are a good match for this position? How would we benefit from hiring you? (See *www.aapa.org/gandp/pro-issues.html#employ*.)

- What were your duties at your previous job? What did you gain from that experience?

- Why did you decide to become a PA?

- What did you do before you became a PA?

- What have you been doing during the time that you have not been working as a PA (if there is a gap in the job seeker's employment history)?

- How do you envision your role in this position? What type of duties do you enjoy most? What do you hope to gain from this position?

- How would you describe yourself? What are your professional interests?

- Where do you see yourself in five years?

- As a supervising physician, what is my liability? How much am I increasing my risk by hiring a PA?

- Do I need to add you to my malpractice insurance, or will you have your own policy?

- Can we bill for your services? Will the income you generate cover your costs to the practice? (See *www.aapa.org/gandp/3rdparty.html#ibs*.)

- How soon could you start working? (You will need a license, malpractice coverage, and possibly hospital privileges before you can work. You should know approximately how long it will take to get those things in place.)

- How much do PAs earn? (See *www.aapa.org/research/index.html* and *www.aapa.org/research/salary.html*.)

QUESTIONS YOU SHOULD ASK THE EMPLOYER

- Have you worked with PAs before? What is your vision of what PAs do?

- What do you know about the PA profession?

- How will you supervise me?

- What hours will I be expected to work?

- What roles will I be expected to play? What would my primary duties be?

- What practice settings would I be working in?

- Do you envision my role or responsibilities changing over time?

- Whose is in charge of scheduling? How will patients be assigned? Who will decide and how? Will I have my own panel of patients?

- How does the telephone triage system work?

- How is the staff structured? Who are the other employees and partners? What are their roles? Who would be available to assist me?

- Is the staff familiar with PAs? Do you plan to educate them on the role of a PA? Is there anything I can do to help?

- How many PAs have been in the position in the past few years?

- Is the practice for sale? Is a sale possible in the next year? Is it merging with a health system?

ANATOMY OF A CONTRACT

The following article outlines basic points to consider in writing an employment contract. More detailed information on contract negotiation can found in AAPA's PA career guide, Contacts and Contracts. You can buy *Contacts and Contracts* by visiting the AAPA On-line Store, *www.aapa.org/aapastore*.

PA compensation plans vary as widely as the multitude of specialties and settings in which PAs practice. Although oral contracts are common, putting all agreements into a written contract protects you if disagreements arise later. The contract should not be written until all parties have agreed on the essential components.

It is advisable to hire a lawyer to review any contract you intend to sign. Retain a lawyer who has knowledge of contracts, particularly health care contracts, and who can help you understand the responsibilities and expectations outlined in the contract. A local lawyer is best; he or she is more likely to be familiar with state and local laws. It also is important to know if the lawyer has handled PA contracts before and how many years of experience he or she has had in the area of contract law.

TERMS AND TERMINATION
The term, or length, of the contract must be stated, including your starting date and the duration of the initial contract. Perhaps more important, the contract should state whether it can be terminated early if notice is given. If so, the amount of notice and reasons for justifying early termination should be carefully described. Termination provisions are either "with cause" or "without cause."

Termination without cause means the contract can be ended by either party at any time without reason. Typically, a 90-day notice is required. You may be able to negotiate for a "balloon buyout" that provides extra compensation.

Termination with cause provisions protect employers from liability due to employees who engage in illegal or illicit behavior. Legitimate causes for dismissal should be clearly defined.

Payment of bonuses, severance pay, and vacation or sick time reimbursement should be addressed. Malpractice insurance premiums should be mentioned to ensure you are not required to refund money your employer has paid for these premiums.

The contract should state how often a formal job performance review will be conducted. For a new position, this is typically at one-month, three-month, and six-month intervals.

CONTRACT RENEWAL
Every contract should include an option to renew or a provision to renegotiate based on a performance evaluation. Performance criteria should be included or attached to the contract.

EMPLOYEE VS. INDEPENDENT CONTRACTOR
State and federal laws vary. It is important to specify the relationship, however, because your employer's liability regarding employment taxes and pension benefits will be affected. The Internal Revenue Service has guidelines that you and your tax advisor should examine.

SERVICES TO BE PROVIDED
The area of medicine in which you practice and your duties and obligations should be clearly defined, including working times, sites, and practice duties. Requirements for rounds and on-call duties should be clearly stated. Be sure to address whether clauses that may prohibit holding a second job apply to volunteer health care or nonmedical employment.

CREDENTIALS AND PRIVILEGES

The contract should specify the professional credentials (for example, NCCPA certification) that you must possess or obtain within a specified time. It also should specify whether you must apply for or obtain privileges at certain hospitals.

COMPENSATION

More disagreements arise over compensation than perhaps any other issue. Will you be paid a salary, an hourly rate, a percentage of fees billed or collected, or salary plus bonus based on productivity? If your compensation will be based on a percentage of fees billed, specify which fees will be included in the calculation. If you will be paid an hourly rate, include a minimum number of hours per week or per month to ensure adequate income.

Terms should be clearly defined in the contract — not only the amount (and/or percentage of productivity income) but also the frequency of calculation and payment. For comparison purposes, find out what colleagues in your area earn from a customized salary profile provided by AAPA for a nominal fee.

MALPRACTICE INSURANCE

Who will pay for malpractice insurance? How much will it cost? Will you be listed on your supervising physician's policy or have your own policy? Be sure to compare the options before you sign the contract.

Become familiar with both occurrence and claims-made policies. An occurrence policy covers alleged negligence that occurs during the policy period, regardless of when claims are reported. Claims-made policies cover incidents that happen and are reported while the policy is in force; for an extra premium, often a large one, tail coverage will protect you against claims filed after the policy ends.

Your malpractice policy should cover liability for services rendered (or not rendered) and all legal costs, regardless of the suit's outcome or whether the suit was fraudulent. Try to obtain an ultimate net-loss policy, which will cover all legal fees.

As a service to its members, AAPA sponsors a professional liability insurance program. For more information and an application form, call 877/356-2272.

FRINGE BENEFITS

The contract should describe both included and excluded fringe benefits. Typical benefits include vacation and education leave, travel expenses related to education leave, professional dues, licensure fees, hospital medical staff fees, books and professional journals, NCCPA fees, Drug Enforcement Administration registration fees, health insurance, disability, life insurance, and retirement plans.

SICK LEAVE AND DISABILITY

The contract should specify if you will continue to be paid if you become sick or disabled, and, if so, for how long. Often practices have different disability policies for physicians and other employees; it is important to understand which one will cover you. If you purchase the policy yourself, the federal government does not tax it; therefore, it may be advantageous for you to do this and negotiate a higher compensation package.

PURCHASING INTO THE PRACTICE

If you hope to buy into the practice eventually, the conditions of the buy-in and basic terms of purchase should be spelled out, usually in a separate letter of intent. This letter should include methods for valuing the practice assets and the physical site, and it should outline your participation in business decisions, the length of time it will take before you become a full partner, and the amount and terms of the purchase.

RESTRICTIVE COVENANTS

A restrictive covenant, sometimes called a "non-compete clause," is a provision in the contract that prohibits you from practicing in a given geographic area or given medical specialty after you leave a practice. This is usually for a defined period of time, often a few years after leaving the practice.

These clauses are enforceable in most states if the terms are considered reasonable. A 10-mile restriction might be reasonable in a rural area but not in a metropolitan area. Consider the following to be red flags for undesirable arrangements: exclusions from practicing in entire countries or states; a prohibition from practicing at a particular hospital; or an employer who says, "Oh, don't worry about signing that; we would never enforce it." If you must negotiate a contract with a restrictive covenant, be sure it is something you can live with. Consider adding a clause that declares the restrictions void if you are dismissed without cause.

DISPUTES

Check that the contract specifies whether disputes between you and your employer will be settled by mandatory arbitration or in court and whether the prevailing party will receive lawyer's fees and costs. The contract also should include a clause that allows you and your lawyer access to patient medical records if a lawsuit is brought against you after you leave the practice. Otherwise, your lawyer may have to subpoena the records, which is a costly process that can take months.

SUMMARY

After meeting with your prospective employer, drafting a contract, reviewing the employee handbook, and discussing the contract with your lawyer, are you ready to sign on the dotted line? Perhaps. As you review each section of the contract, imagine situations that could arise. Ask yourself, "What would happen if...?" Then make your decision based on a knowledge-able review of the contract and good common sense.

CONTRACT CHECKLIST

DEFINING YOUR DUTIES – HAVE YOU

☐ Received a copy of the employee handbook?

☐ Defined the term of the contract?

☐ Defined the number of days of notice that must be given prior to terminations?

☐ Defined whether you will be an employee or an independent contractor?

☐ If independent contractor, met with your tax advisor to review tax implications?

☐ Clearly defined duties and work hours?

☐ Discussed with the employer whether various third-party payer contracts include compensation for services provided by a PA?

_____

_____

_____

_____

_____

_____

_____

_____

_____

_____

_____

BENEFITS – HAVE YOU

☐ Determined the amount of compensation?

☐ If paid a percentage of revenue, agreed on how it will be calculated?

☐ Defined whether the employer will pay for NCCPA certification/recertification, licensing fees, hospital medical staff fees, and DEA registration fees, if applicable?

☐ Are health and dental insurance provided? Does employer pay the full premium(s)? Is it single or family coverage?

☐ Is life insurance provided? How much coverage? Does employer pay the full premium?

☐ Is disability provided? What is the elimination period, length of time you may be disabled, and amount of disability income you will receive? Do you have the option of paying the premium to avoid taxes on the benefit?

☐ Is malpractice insurance provided? Limits of coverage? Is tail or nose coverage provided? Is it your own policy or are you covered under an umbrella or a rider? Do you have a copy?

☐ How much paid time off for CME, vacation, holidays, and sick leave?

☐ Is maternity/paternity leave provided?

☐ Can you participate in pension and profit-sharing plans?

☐ Are funds available for CME fees and travel?

☐ Are AAPA and state chapter dues paid by employer?

☐ Are relocation and interview expenses reimbursed?

☐ Agreed on the timing of performance reviews?

_____

_____

_____

_____

_____

_____

_____

_____

_____

_____

_____

_____

LEGAL ISSUES

☐ Is a restrictive convenant included in the contract? If so, do you understand its legal ramifications?

☐ Has your lawyer reviewed the contract?

_____

_____

_____

_____

_____

_____

_____

BEFORE YOU MAKE YOUR DECISION

AAPA recommends utilizing this checklist to assist you with analyzing your employment options when beginning your job search. Ask these questions and get satisfactory answers before making an employment decision.

Practice Issues

HOURS AND LOCATION

☐ How many office locations are there? How many of these will you be expected to work in?
☐ What are the hours of operation for each location?
☐ How many hours of work are expected per week?
☐ Is there an on-call schedule? Is it flexible?
☐ How will holidays be covered?
☐ What time do weekends begin and end?

RESPONSIBILITIES

☐ Is this the type of work you want to do?
☐ What are the physician's expectations of what you will do?
☐ How will you and the supervising physician interact? How will supervision be provided?
☐ What is the availability of the supervising physician?
☐ What is your relationship to others in the office? Will you have any supervisory responsibilities?
☐ In how many hospitals is the physician privileged? Will you be privileged there, too?
☐ What are your hospital responsibilities (rounds, ER, evaluations, deliveries, surgical assisting)?
☐ Is hospital committee work a possibility?
☐ In how many nursing homes does the physician follow patients?
☐ What will be your responsibilities in the nursing homes?

LEGAL ISSUES

☐ Is the necessary paperwork filed with state licensing board or department?
☐ Are the state statute and regulations reviewed with the physician?
☐ Are the rules/regulations and "gray areas" discussed?
☐ Are the nursing home regulations reviewed?
☐ Is there a probationary period?
☐ Is a written contract provided?
☐ Are the physician's malpractice policy type and coverage reviewed and discussed?
☐ Are the PA's malpractice policy type and coverage discussed and acquired?
☐ Is tail coverage provided, if needed?

Business/Benefits

INSURANCE

☐ What is the malpractice coverage (personal occurrence policy, personal claims-made policy with paid tail coverage, or rider on physician's policy)?
☐ Is health insurance provided? For dependents?
☐ Is dental insurance provided? For dependents?
☐ Is life insurance provided?
☐ Is disability insurance provided?

LEAVE

☐ What is the annual leave policy?
☐ What are the paid holidays?
☐ What is the sick leave policy?
☐ What is the family/maternity leave policy?
☐ What is the unpaid leave policy?
☐ How many days are given for paid jury duty?
☐ How many days are given for CME?

PROFESSIONAL EXPENSES

☐ Is the PANCE expense covered?
☐ Is the PANRE expense covered?
☐ Is AAPA's annual conference expense covered?
☐ Are state chapter CME conference expenses covered?
☐ What amount is available for CME?
☐ Are AAPA annual membership dues covered?
☐ Are the state chapter annual membership dues covered?
☐ Is professional activity in local, state, and national PA organizations permitted?
☐ Is malpractice insurance paid/provided?

INCOME

☐ What is the base salary? Is this in line with your salary survey findings?
☐ Is a partnership available?
☐ How often will you be paid?
☐ How often will you receive a performance review?
☐ Is there a bonus plan available?
☐ Is there a profit-sharing plan available?
☐ Is a pension provided?

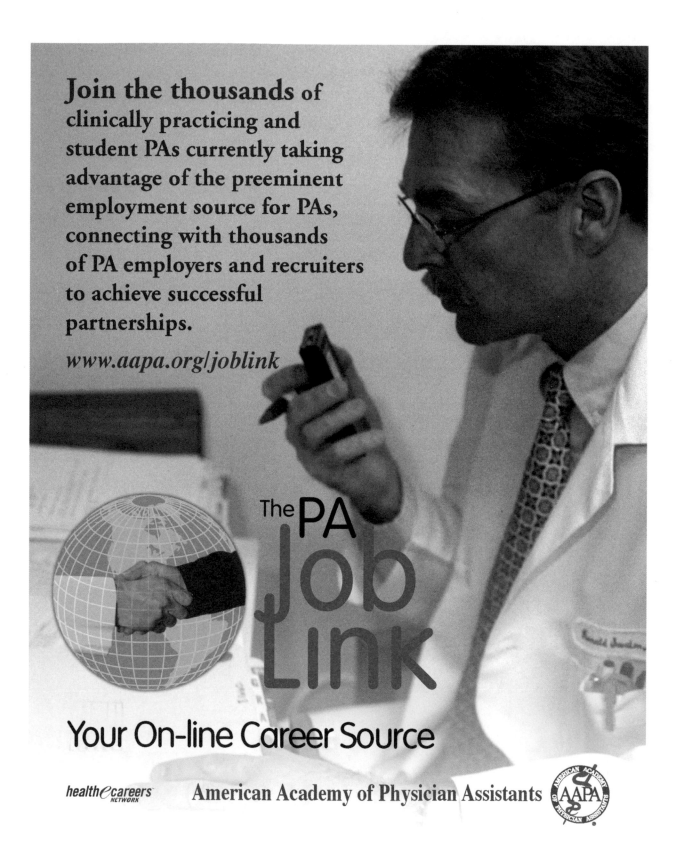

Section III

What You Need to Know —
Professional Issues

ESTABLISHING A PROFESSIONAL FILE

A professional file is a record of your education, career, professional materials, and achievements that you maintain continuously throughout your career. This reference will be important when you apply for employment or licensure, enroll for postgraduate training, submit your continuing medical education hours, submit a manuscript for publications, etc., as all of the requested information will be already gathered together and located in a safe place.

It is important to begin establishing a professional file while you are still a student so that you have all your records from your education as well as the information from the beginning of your career as a practicing PA, and so you get in the habit of maintaining a professional file.

Every professional file is different as everyone's path after graduation and certification varies; therefore there is no comprehensive list of items to include in a professional file; however, there are many materials which should be collected and maintained by all PAs. These are listed below.

- **Transcripts and diplomas:** Maintain a copy of each, even though you might need to request official transcripts later.

- **Clinical rotation information:** Location, dates, names, and positions of people worked with, contact information for preceptor worked with, and duties performed on rotation for each of your rotations

- **Résumé and curriculum vitae (CV):** Always have these up-to-date and ready to submit, so that you do not miss out on an opportunity because it takes you several days to piece together a current one.

- **References:** Professional references are important, so anticipate those that will be most helpful and request them early before the reference is needed. If someone volunteers to provide a reference "in case you ever need one," accept it and then keep it on file.

- **Personal correspondence:** Maintain congratulatory letters and endorsements from patients or agencies you may have assisted. These often become the basis for more formal references in the future. This might also include newspaper articles featuring you or your practice or information brochures produced for patient education.

- **Licensing/registration/certification materials:** Keep a copy of your license or documentation of your registration in your state. Also maintain copies of your credentials from various trainings you may have completed (BLS, ACLS, PALS, ATLS, etc.).

- **CME records:** In addition to your NCCPA records, keep a copy of the CME logging form and certificates of completion from all CME courses you attend. In the event of an audit by your state or NCCPA, this documentation will be required.

- **Malpractice insurance records:** Keep copies of all policies you currently hold and any that you held in the past.

- **Publications:** File copies of any articles that your author or co-author, as well as any reviews or correspondence referencing the article or paper.

- **Expense record:** Keep receipts for all professional dues, expenses related to your practice, equipment you bought for your practice, CME expenses, etc. Whether deducting on your taxes or requesting reimbursement from your employer, you will need receipts when it is time to file.

- **Procedure log:** Hospitals frequently credential and privilege PAs in the same way they credential and privilege physicians. Some will require documentation of previous experience before granting some privileges. The log should include the name of institution, type of procedure, date, and the supervising physician's name.

- **Organization record:** For any professional organization that you belong to, keep records of your membership, positions of leadership you held, meeting you attended, and activities which you were involved in with the organization.

- **Award or honors:** Keep track of any awards or honors that you receive as a professional.

PRE-PRACTICE CHECKLIST

YOU HAVE GRADUATED, ACCEPTED A JOB, AND ARE READY TO BEGIN PRACTICE. SO WHAT IS NEEDED PRIOR TO YOUR FIRST DAY OF WORK?

Here is a checklist of items that you might need to work as a practicing physician assistant.

☐ State license (in most states, a new graduate license is available for the time period between graduation and receiving the results of PANCE, *www.aapa.org/gandp/temprov.html*): *www.aapa.org/gandp/statereg.html*

☐ NCCPA certification: *www.nccpa.net*

☐ Medicare Provider Identification Number: *www.cms.hhs.gov* or from local Medicare Part B carrier, *www.cms.hhs.gov/contacts/incardir.asp#1*

☐ Medicaid provider number (if required in your state): *www.cms.hhs.gov/medicaid/allStateContacts.asp*

☐ Provider numbers for private insurance companies accepted at your practice or authorization to bill under your supervising physician's provider number if the company does not give numbers to PAs

☐ Malpractice insurance: *www.aapa.org/gandp/risky.html* or *www.epreceptor.com/aapa_insurance/index.html*

☐ DEA number (if prescribing controlled substances): *www.deadiversion.usdoj.gov/*

☐ State controlled substance number (required in some states): *www.aapa.org/gandp/statereg.html*

☐ Delegation agreement or any other state-required agreement with your supervising physician: *www.aapa.org/gandp/statelaw.html*

☐ Hospital privileges: *www.aapa.org/gandp/pro-issues.html#hospital*

☐ Copy of state statue and administrative rules that govern practice from your state licensing board: *www.aapa.org/gandp/statereg.html*

☐ Copy of everything in your professional file, saved in a safe place

The above checklist is a good resource not only for your first job as a PA, but for every job you may hold as a clinically practicing PA. You may find you are not required to have every item on the list (for example, you do not need hospital privileges if you will never see patients in a hospital setting), but you do need to think about each of these items and how it relates to the laws in your state and the job you are about to begin.

You can find additional information about the items on the checklist throughout this publication and also on AAPA's Web site (*www.aapa.org*).

PROFESSIONAL RESOURCE SERIES

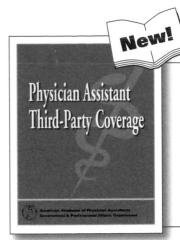

Physician Assistant Third-Party Coverage

This excellent resource summarizes third-party coverage policies for PA medical and surgical services, and outlines rules, regulations, and billing concepts for coverage of physician services provided by PAs under Medicare, Medicaid, TRICARE/CHAMPUS, and private insurance companies. Practical issues such as strategies for handling claim denials are also covered. This book provides the physician assistant with insight into courses of action that can be taken to help solve problems and maintain a more positive reimbursement environment. (140 pages)

Item #112   Member: $25.00   Nonmember: $50.00

Hiring a Physician Assistant

This book is an invaluable resource for employers who have hired PAs before and for those exploring the idea for the first time. It can also serve as an excellent job search tool to use with prospective employers. Included is information about educational requirements for physician assistants, guidelines regarding their scope of responsibilities and practice, and a pre-employment checklist. The book also covers topics such as state regulations, national certification, malpractice coverage, employment agreements, recruiting, and compensation. (68 pages)

Item #152   Member: $25.00   Nonmember: $50.00

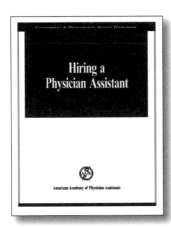

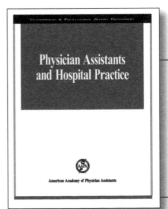

Physician Assistants and Hospital Practice

Formerly titled *Hospital Privileges,* this publication is a summary of information on the practice of PAs in hospitals. It contains policy statements from national organizations, information about JCAHO, patient restraints, EMTALA, model hospital bylaws, and a sample credentialing form. This book is perfect for medical staff administrators and PAs seeking information about employing and utilizing physician assistants. (74 pages)

Item #106   Member: $25.00   Nonmember: $50.00

Save 20% when you purchase all three titles in the series

Item #F155   Member: $60.00   Nonmember: $120.00

Prices subject to change.

Section IV

WHAT YOU NEED TO KNOW —
STATE LAWS
& REGULATIONS

STATE LAWS

Successful completion of your physician assistant education is an important milestone in your career as a PA. Now you are ready to start putting all those clinical skills to work.

To use your new education, you will need to be authorized to practice by the state in which you are going to work. State laws and regulations dictate who may practice as a PA, the medical services a PA may perform, and the requirements for supervision. State PA laws also contain sections defining the responsibilities of the regulatory board and disciplinary actions that may be taken against PAs who have violated the law.

Every state has a unique set of requirements and procedures. Most states grant "licenses" to physician assistants. However, some states use the terms "registration" or "certification" for PAs who are authorized to practice in the state. Forty-eight states plus the District of Columbia and Guam allow physicians to delegate prescriptive authority to PAs.

Of particular importance to new graduates is the section in most state laws that deals with "temporary" or "graduate" licensure. This category is created to allow new PA graduates to practice between graduation and NCCPA certification. Laws in 44 states allow new graduates to practice with "temporary" or "graduate" licenses. One additional state (Colorado) has no temporary or graduate classification but allows precertified PAs to practice under special provisions. The District of Columbia does not permit PAs to be licensed prior to NCCPA certification. Some states require more direct supervision or a more limited scope of practice (i.e., no prescribing) for graduate or temporary licensees. You must apply for a temporary or graduate license just as you do for full licensure and you may not work as a PA until it is issued.

> **You must apply for a temporary or graduate license just as you do for full licensure and you may not work as a PA until it is issued.**

Most state laws dictate that temporary or graduate licenses are valid only until NCCPA exam scores are available. At that time, you need to contact the licensing agency to convert to full licensure status if you pass the exam or to inquire about an extended temporary license if you do not. Only a handful of states will extend a temporary or graduate license for PAs who do not pass the NCCPA exam.

It is the responsibility of each PA to make sure that you have a valid and current state license (or registration or certification, as the case may be) and have met any additional state requirements before you begin to practice. Once you've started working, it is your responsibility to ensure that everything you do is within the limits of your state law and regulations. To obtain an application for licensure, or for more specific information, contact the PA licensing agency in the state where you are planning to practice.

Approximately 10 percent of PAs are employed by the federal government. Each federal employer of PAs (such as the Department of Veterans Affairs, Indian Health Service, Federal Bureau of Prisons, and the military) has its own requirements for PA practice. If you plan to work for a branch of the federal government, it is your responsibility to make sure that you are appropriately credentialed by your federal employer before you begin to work.

Some new graduates find the language in state law or the process itself to be confusing. AAPA can help. We have summaries of state laws and summaries of legal requirements for new graduates. The document that describes graduate or temporary license requirements in a state-by-state format is entitled Summary of Provisions Regarding New Graduate Licensure. It is available on the AAPA Web Site at *www.aapa.org/gandp/temprov.html.*

PARTICIPATING IN CARE DURING DISASTERS AND EMERGENCIES

The AAPA Guidelines for Ethical Conduct and the normal human compassionate response call for physician assistants to care for patients in emergency situations. However, it can be difficult to be an ad hoc volunteer in the case of disasters and emergencies. Many different laws govern the situation, some of which are difficult to know about in advance.

If you think you're going to want to volunteer in the future, join an organized disaster response program now. Otherwise, check the AAPA Web site for current information during a disaster such as Hurricane Katrina.

SUMMARY CHART
STATE STATUTORY AND REGULATORY REQUIREMENTS FOR LICENSURE

State	Graduation from PA Program	Passage of NCCPA Exam (PANCE)	Current NCCPA Certification	New Graduate Authorization	Renewal Requirements	Prescribing Privileges
Alabama	•	•		•	CME	•
Alaska	•	•	•	•	NCCPA	•
Arizona	•	•	•	•	CME	•
Arkansas	• *and bachelor's degree*	•		•	CME	•
California	•	•		•		•
Colorado	•	•		*		•
Connecticut	• *and bachelor's degree*	•	•	•	NCCPA	•
Delaware	•	•		•	CME	•
District of Columbia	•	•			CME	•
Florida	•	•		•	CME	•
Osteopathic	•	•		•	*CME*	•
Georgia	•	•		•	CME	•
Hawaii	•	•	•	•	NCCPA	•
Idaho	• *and bachelor's degree*	•		•	CME	•
Illinois		•	•	•	NCCPA	•
Indiana	•	•	•	•	NCCPA	
Iowa	•	•		•	CME	•
Kansas	•	•		•	CME	•
Kentucky	•	•		•	NCCPA	•
Louisiana	•	•	•	•	NCCPA	•
Maine	• *and/or*	•		•	CME	•
Osteopathic	• *and/or*	•		•	*CME*	•
Maryland	• *and bachelor's degree*	•		•	CME	•
Massachusetts	• *and bachelor's degree*	•		•	CME	•
Michigan	•	•		•		•
Osteopathic	•	•		•		•
Minnesota		•	•	•	CME (NCCPA for Rx)	•
Mississippi	• *and master's degree*	•	•	•	CME	•

State	Graduation from PA Program	Passage of NCCPA Exam (PANCE)	Current NCCPA Certification	New Graduate Authorization	Renewal Requirements	Prescribing Privileges
Missouri	**	•	•	•	NCCPA	•
Montana	•	•	•		NCCPA	•
Nebraska	•	•		•	CME	•
Nevada	•	•	•	•	NCCPA	•
Osteopathic	•	•	•	•	*CME*	•
New Hampshire	•	•	•		NCCPA	•
New Jersey	•	•		•	CME	•
New Mexico	•	•	•	•	NCCPA	•
Osteopathic	•	•	•		*NCCPA*	•
New York	•	•		•		•
North Carolina	•	•			CME	•
North Dakota		•	•		NCCPA	•
Ohio		•	•	•	NCCPA	•
Oklahoma	•	•			CME	•
Oregon	•	•		•	NCCPA for Sch. II prescribing	•
Pennsylvania	• *and bachelor's degree*	•	•	•	NCCPA	•
Osteopathic	•	•	•		*NCCPA*	
Rhode Island	•	•		•	CME	•
South Carolina	•	•	•	•	NCCPA	•
South Dakota	•	•		•	CME	•
Tennessee	•	•		•	CME	•
Texas	•	•	•	•	CME	•
Utah	•	•		•	CME	•
Vermont	•	•		•	CME	•
Virginia	•	•	•	•	NCCPA	•
Washington	•	•		•	CME	•
Osteopathic	•	•		•	*CME (NCCPA for Rx)*	•
West Virginia	•	•	•	•	CME (NCCPA for Rx)	•
Osteopathic	•	•	•	•	*CME (NCCPA for Rx)*	•
Wisconsin	•	•	•	•		•
Wyoming	•	•	•	•	NCCPA	•

December 2005

* *New graduates may practice under supervising physician's delegatory authority with direct supervision.*

** *Program requirement waived for those employed as PAs prior to 1986.*

WORKING INTERNATIONALLY

There are avenues for PAs to practice internationally, although a PA who wishes to work abroad may have to do some sleuthing to find the right opportunity. PAs encounter challenges in arranging to work abroad that they do not face stateside. The first challenge is that the PA profession is not widely recognized outside the United States. Some countries have health care providers similar to American PAs or are in the process of developing the profession. In general, however, there are no set standards of education, licensing, or reciprocity for PAs to work in other countries. In 2002 the Province of Manitoba, Canada, passed enabling legislation to allow organizations to hire American PAs; however, there are no reciprocity laws enabling Canadian PAs to work in the U.S. PAs also now work in the United Kingdom, and have been able to practice under the general delegatory clause of the British Medical Act. PAs interested in job opportunities should keep their eyes open for ads in *AAPA News*, *JAAPA*, and The PA Job Link.

LICENSURE AND LIABILITY COVERAGE

PAs may also face questions about physician supervision and liability coverage. AAPA's Guidelines for PAs Working Internationally, approved by the 2001 House of Delegates, state that PAs must establish the appropriate physician-PA team. That can be done with an American physician or local physician in the country. Because there are no licensing laws or practice acts for PAs working abroad, special arrangements have to be made through the ministry of health of the host country. In the case of U.S. corporations with international sites, you may find the company falling back on the licensing laws of the state in which their headquarters are located. Licensing issues also raise questions about physician supervision of PAs. Problems may arise if the physician and the PA are licensed by different states. Liability insurers may have other requirements and obligations for insureds who are outside the jurisdiction of U.S. courts.

Many insurance companies will not cover PAs outside the U.S., so it is important to contact your carrier prior to leaving the country. It is important to explore and resolve these types of issues before working abroad.

The most up-to-date information on international employment and volunteer opportunities for physician assistants can be found on AAPA's International PA Development Web page, *www.aapa.org/international/index.html*. There you will find information on international practice, ethical guidelines, as well as numerous resources and links.

Also available on the page is a link to a database of PAs who will share stories and information about their work in specific countries. PAs who have worked internationally can add their names to the database through a link on the page.

For PA students interested in setting up their own international rotations, the page offers information to help you get started, as well as links to other organizations that may be helpful.

If you're already planning a trip, the page offers a checklist of items and information you should obtain before setting off on your journey.

For more information about the international resources AAPA offers, contact Marie-Michele Leger at *mleger@aapa.org*.

GUIDELINES FOR PAs WORKING INTERNATIONALLY

POLICY OF THE AMERICAN ACADEMY OF PHYSICIAN ASSISTANTS

1. PAs should establish and maintain the appropriate physician-PA team.

2. PAs should accurately represent their skills, training, professional credentials, identity, or service both directly and indirectly.

3. PAs should provide only those services for which they are qualified via their education and/or experiences, and in accordance with all pertinent legal and regulatory processes.

4. PAs should respect the culture, values, beliefs, and expectations of the patients, local health care providers, and the local health care systems.

5. PAs should take responsibility for being familiar with, and adhering to the customs, laws, and regulations of the country where they will be providing services.

6. When applicable, PAs should identify and train local personnel who can assume the role of providing care and continuing the education process.

H-P-3700.3.1: Guidelines for PAs Working Internationally, adopted 2001.

Section V

What You Need to Know —
Certification &
Recertification

LICENSURE VS. CERTIFICATION: WHAT IS THE DIFFERENCE?

Licensure is a requirement that authorizes you to practice as a physician assistant providing patient services and is issued by the state in which you plan to work.

Certification is voluntary, except as it may be required by your state licensing board and is conferred by the National Commission on Certification of Physician Assistants (NCCPA). See the chart on page 28 for individual state certification requirements.

HOW TO GET LICENSED
PANCE — The Initial Exam
To become licensed, you must successfully pass the Physician Assistant National Certifying Examination (PANCE). The exam is administered by the NCCPA at more than 300 Prometric Testing Centers throughout the country and is offered during four overlapping administrations each year. You will need to contact NCCPA for details on when and how to register for the exam. The best way to obtain information about PANCE is to visit NCCPA's Web site at *www.nccpa.net* or phone 678/417-8100.

PREPARING FOR PANCE
You should apply for PANCE before you graduate, but you must have completed all requirements for graduation before you can actually take the exam. AAPA has assembled a comprehensive list of exam review resources to help you prepare for the PANCE exam. The list includes publications (with ordering information), review courses (with contact names and phone numbers so you can register), and one on-line review course. Go to *www.aapa.org/cme/index.html#exam* for complete details.

CONTACT YOUR STATE LICENSING BOARD
Before you take the PANCE, you should contact the state licensing board where you plan to obtain complete information on how to apply for your first state license. Contact information for all state licensing boards can be found on page 93 of this publication or on-line at *www.aapa.org/gandp/statereg. html.*

HOW TO RENEW YOUR LICENSE
Although all 50 states require that you pass the PANCE to obtain initial licensure, license renewal requirements vary by state. Some states require that you maintain NCCPA certification for license renewal while others require that you earn CME only. Five states require neither CME nor NCCPA certification to renew your state license. All PAs should obtain a copy of the statute and administrative rules that govern their state license. Contact information for state licensing boards can be found on page 93 of this publication. Please refer to the chart above right for your state's license renewal requirements.

RENEWAL REQUIREMENTS VARY BY STATE

27 states require CME	AL, AZ, AR, DE, DC, FL, GA, ID, IA, KS, ME, MD, MA, MN*, MS, NE, NJ, NC, OK, RI, SD, TN, TX, UT, VT, WA*, WV*
18 states require NCCPA certification	AK, CT, HI, IL, IN, KY, LA, MO, MT, NV**, NH, NM, ND, OH, PA, SC, VA, WY
1 state requires NCCPA certification to prescribe Schedule II	OR
3 states require NCCPA certification for license renewal with Rx privileges	MN*, WA*, WV*
5 states have no CME requirements for license renewal	CA, CO, MI, NY, WI

*Note inclusion in two categories

**The Osteopathic Licensing Board in Nevada requires CME only.

CME REQUIREMENTS VARY BY STATE
Eleven states have topic-specific CME requirements for license renewal (see chart on page 34). In most cases, this means that the designated number of CME hours must be earned during each license renewal period. To assist AAPA members in meeting these requirements, the Topic-specific CME Series was developed. For complete information about the Topic-specific CME Series, see details on page 34.

TOPIC-SPECIFIC CME REQUIREMENTS BY STATE

State	Specific CME Requirement
Florida	1 hour domestic violence, 1 hour in HIV/AIDS (courses in palliative or end-of-life care may be substituted), 2 hours in prevention of medical errors. Prescribing PAs must complete a minimum of 10 hours of CME in specialty area of supervising physician biennially (these hours may apply toward 100-hour requirement).
Georgia	3 hours in practice-specific pharmaceuticals
Kentucky	2 hours in HIV/AIDS
Maryland	PAs must complete a course on the needs of the terminally ill for recertification.
Massachusetts	At least 4 hours of required CME must be in pharmacology or pharmacokinetics.
Nevada	4 hours in the medical consequences of an act of terrorism that involves the use of a weapon of mass destruction. PAs attending a CME class on geriatrics and gerontology are entitled to receive twice the hours actually spent in the course.
Oklahoma	1 hour every year on the topic of substance abuse
South Dakota	Renewal request must be accompanied by proof of 30 postgraduate hours in family medicine approved by the board within 12 months.
Texas	Board may grant exemption of up to half of the 40 hours required CME if a PA provides volunteer services at a site serving medically underserved population, other than the site of the license holder's primary practice.
Washington	At least 7 clock hours of AIDS education and training are required for renewal.
West Virginia	To maintain prescribing privileges, a PA must complete 10 hours of CME in rational drug therapy in each certification period.

HOW TO GET CERTIFIED

National certification is conferred by the National Commission on Certification of Physician Assistants (NCCPA), an independent agency formed by 14 organizations in 1975. NCCPA is responsible for the administration of all nationally recognized physician assistant examinations.

To obtain additional information on certification, visit the NCCPA Web site at *www.nccpa.net* or phone 678/417-8100.

PHYSICIAN ASSISTANT NATIONAL CERTIFYING EXAMINATION

To obtain initial NCCPA certification, a PA must successfully complete the Physician Assistant National Certifying Examination (PANCE). PANCE is designed to assess general medical and surgical knowledge and is administered by computer at testing centers throughout the country during four testing windows each year. After passing PANCE, physician assistants are issued an NCCPA certificate, entitling them to use of the PA-C designation until the expiration date printed on the certificate (approximately two years).

ELIGIBILITY FOR PANCE

Before taking PANCE, a candidate must have graduated, or completed the requirements for graduation, from a physician assistant program or surgeon assistant program accredited by the Accreditation Review Commission on Education for the Physician Assistant (ARC-PA). Candidates who have been awarded unrestricted eligibility by NCCPA under earlier policies are also eligible for the exam.

HOW TO MAINTAIN YOUR CERTIFICATION

National certification for physician assistants is voluntary except as required by certain states for licensure (see the chart on page 28) or otherwise by your employer. To maintain a valid NCCPA certificate, PAs must complete an ongoing six-year process of certification maintenance that involves CME logging and a recertification exam.

Step 1: CME Logging – every two years

Every two years, a minimum of 100 hours of CME credit must be earned including at least 50 hours of Category I (Preapproved) credit.

Category I activities are preapproved because they have been reviewed by one of the following organizations: AAPA, organizations accredited by ACCME (including AMA), AAFP, or AOACCME (see Table 1 on page 35.) All Category I activities must be documented with certificates of completion or attendance or some other official verification from the program's provider. All documentation for Category I activities should be retained in your professional file for seven years in case you are audited.

CME requirement: 50 hours

Category II activities are elective; they have not been reviewed for educational content. Category II activities should be chosen according to the following guidelines and submitted on an hour-per-hour basis:

- Any practice related program that is not eligible for Category I (Preapproved) CME credit. This includes many educational programs provided by pharmaceutical companies and medical device manufacturers.

- Any practice related, voluntary, self-learning activity, e.g., journal reading, medical text reading, precepting

- Any practice-related postgraduate course, excluding courses taken in an actual PA program

CME requirement: There are none. Category II activities are optional.

All hours must be earned by June 30 of the certificate expiration year. See Table 2.

ACCEPTABLE CATEGORY I CME

CE, CEU, and CEH credits are not acceptable for Category I CME. The PA profession is based on the physician model, and PAs may only submit CME credits in fulfillment of their Category I requirement. Category I (Preapproved) CME credit may be submitted from programs approved and designated according to Table 1.

Table 1
Organizations That Approve CME Which Can Be Submitted as Category I Credit by Physician Assistants

Sponsor (organization approving CME credit)	Credit Designation
American Academy of Physician Assistants (AAPA)	Category I
American Osteopathic Association Council on Continuing Medical Education (AOACCME)	Category I
American Academy of Family Physicians (AAFP)	Prescribed Credit
Organizations accredited by the Accreditation Council on Continuing Medical Education (ACCME). The The American Medical Association (AMA) is part of this group.	AMA Category I credit for the Physician's Recognition Award (PRA)

HOW TO SUBMIT CME HOURS FOR NCCPA CERTIFICATION

All CME hours must be submitted on-line or by mail to NCCPA. Please see Table 2 for logging deadlines. Table 3 gives you logging fees and submission addresses.

Table 2
Expiration Year Logging Deadlines*
Deadlines and fees are subject to change. Visit *www.nccpa.net* for the most current requirements.

Last date to earn CME without penalty	June 30
Transition months (CME may apply toward either beginning or ending cycle)	May-June
Begin earning CME for next cycle as early as	May 1
$100 penalty to NCCPA if CME postmark or on-line submission after	June 30
Certificate expires and final deadline	Dec 31

* *If you are submitting CME hours for the first time, please contact NCCPA for deadlines, which may vary depending on when your certificate was issued.*

Table 3
Logging Fees and Submission Address

	Address	Fee
By mail	12000 Findley Road, Suite 200, Duluth, GA 30097	$95
On-line	*www.nccpa.net*	$80

Step 2. Recertification — every six years

To maintain NCCPA certification, a PA must pass either PANRE or Pathway II before the expiration date at the end of the sixth year of the certification maintenance cycle. Either exam may be taken as early as year five, and with multiple exam windows each year, a PA could have as many as four opportunities (two per year) to take and pass a recertification exam.

PANRE is a computer-based exam administered at Prometric testing centers throughout the country.

Pathway II is an alternative to PANRE and involves completing an elective component requirement prior to receiving a Web-based, take-home exam. The elective component involves earning 100 points within the following categories.

Elective Component Categories

- Category I CME
- Clinical skills training
- Medical teaching
- Publications
- Postgraduate coursework
- Professionally relevant postgraduate degree
- Specialty review
- Other

Elective component activities may be completed at any time during the current six-year NCCPA certificate maintenance cycle. (PAs must also complete the 100-hour CME requirement for each CME logging cycle within the NCCPA certification maintenance cycle. Programs and activities used for the CME logging requirement may not also be used for the elective component requirement of Pathway II.) After the elective component has been completed, a PA is eligible for the Web-based, take-home examination, which may be completed with the aid of references.

For complete details about Pathway II, visit NCCPA's Web site, *www.nccpa.net*.

Questions about PANRE or Pathway II should be directed to NCCPA at 678/417-8100 or *nccpa@nccpa.net*.

CME FOR CERTIFICATION AND LICENSURE

Both national certification and state licensure require a commitment to lifelong learning: continuing medical education (CME). AAPA helps you meet that commitment by making sure that you have access to more than enough CME to meet the requirements of your state licensing board and/or national certification.

WHEN SHOULD YOU BEGIN EARNING CME CREDIT?

You should not start earning CME credit until the issuance date on your NCCPA certificate. Many PA students are eager to begin earning CME credit and attend conferences right after they graduate. That is great and you should enjoy the learning, camaraderie, and networking opportunities with your health care colleagues. But please remember that CME credits will not count toward your first logging cycle until the issuance date on your NCCPA certificate.

CME OPPORTUNITIES

AAPA's Annual Conference

AAPA's Annual PA Conference offers five-and-a-half days of CME. With multiple sessions running concurrently, there is a session to meet every need. And with input from AAPA's specialty organizations, caucuses, and special interest groups, topics range from dermatology to cardiology, from sports injuries to palliative medicine, and everything in between. Some sessions are geared for new PAs grads, and the instructional level is basic; other sessions are planned for the more experienced practitioner, and the instructional level is intermediate or advanced. While a PA may earn up to 45-50 hours of Category I CME by attending a session during every time block, most PAs comfortably earn 30-35 CME credits and still find time to network with colleagues and enjoy the host city. For information on AAPA's 34th Annual PA Conference, scheduled for May 27-June 1 in San Francisco, go to *www.aapa.org*.

Athletic Trainer Credit: AAPA is an approved provider of continuing education activities by the National Athletic Trainers' Association Board of Certification (NATABOC). This is an important service for those who maintain dual certification as a PA and an athletic trainer. AAPA's 2005 annual conference in Orlando included approximately 150 sessions that were designated for athletic trainer credit as well as CME credit of PAs. Future annual conferences, including the 2006 conference in San Francisco, will include sessions designated for NATABOC credit as well as CME credit for PAs.

State PA Conferences

Many state organizations hold one or two conferences each year, and AAPA works closely with their leaders to make sure that these state meetings qualify for Category I CME as well. For a complete listing of upcoming state conferences, go to *www.aapa.org/cme/approvedcat1.html*.

The Journal of the American Academy of Physician Assistants (JAAPA) and *AAPA News* also include a listing of CME conferences, but because of space limitations, these listings are not as comprehensive as the one on the Web site.

Local CME Groups

Many states have regional chapters or affiliates to allow members to attend short CME meetings close to home. With careful adherence to AAPA's Standards for Commercial Support, many of these regional CME meetings also receive a Category I (Preapproved) CME credit designation. Most of these CME opportunities are announced locally only. Information on local CME groups can be obtained from your state's constituent organization.

HOME STUDY

Enduring Materials

Home Study Programs (enduring materials) enable PAs to earn Category I CME without leaving home. They are offered in a variety of formats, including monographs, CD-ROMs, Web-based programs, audio- and videotapes and audio- and video-conferences. Category I CME credit is awarded with the successful completion of a post-test. For a complete listing of home study programs, go to *www.aapa.org/cme/index.html* and look for the link to Home Study Programs. The list of offerings is constantly changing, but currently, more than 50 hours of Category I CME can be earned through AAPA-approved home study. Most home study programs are available at no charge for AAPA fellow members, although a few programs do have a registration fee.

Of special note is a two-hour home study program on Patient Communication and Adverse Outcomes that allows you to earn a 10 percent discount on your AAPA-endorsed malpractice insurance (70% score required). A registration fee is required.

JAAPA

Each month, *JAAPA* offers one hour of Category I CME credit based on two or three articles in the current issue. This service is free to AAPA fellow members who can submit the post-test on-line and receive their certificate immediately, or mail it in and receive a certificate within four to six weeks. Nonmembers may submit the post-test by mail along with a $20 scoring fee.

Topic-specific CME

This series of audiotapes was developed to assist PAs meet license renewal requirements in the 11 states that have topic-specific CME requirements. Pharmacology, domestic violence, HIV/AIDS, bioterrorism, and prevention of medical errors are a few of the topics with a specific credit-hour requirement for licensure renewal in some states.

The audiotapes are recordings of CME sessions presented during one of AAPA's recent annual conferences. To keep the series current, new titles are added each year while older ones expire. Successful completion of a post-test (70% minimum score) is required to earn CME credit.

This very cost-effective service is for AAPA fellow members only. (Most titles cost just $5). AAPA student members who are applying for licensure in states that require documentation of topic-specific instruction for initial licensure should contact AAPA at 703/836-2272, ext. 3350, for special assistance. For a current listing of available titles and ordering instructions, go to *www.aapa.org/cme/index.html*.

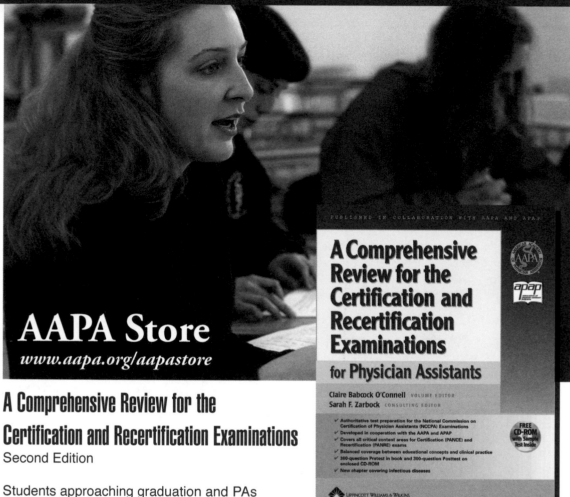

Section VI

What You Need to Know —
Third-Party Reimbursement

OVERVIEW: THIRD-PARTY REIMBURSEMENT

AAPA's Government and Professional Affairs Department is dedicated to assuring that physician assistants are appropriately covered and reimbursed under the Medicare program. The information below has been compiled by AAPA to assist PAs who treat Medicare patients. For additional information related to Medicare coverage, visit AAPA's Web site *(www.aapa.org)* under reimbursement on the professional issues list or view the Centers for Medicare and Medicaid Services Web site *(www. cms.hhs.gov/)*. You can also contact AAPA Government and Professional Affairs staff with your questions.

MEDICARE PROVIDER ELIGIBILITY
For a physician assistant to be an eligible Medicare provider, he or she must meet the following requirements:
- Have graduated from an accredited physician assistant education program, **or**
- Have passed the national certification examination administered by the National Commission on Certification of Physician Assistants (NCCPA), **and**
- Be licensed (authorized) by the state to practice as a physician assistant

MEDICARE PAYMENT POLICY
Effective January 1, 1998, Medicare covers services provided by PAs in all practice settings at a uniform rate of 85 percent of the physician fee schedule, with scope of practice and supervision determined by state law. Services should be billed at the physician rate under the PA's provider number. Medicare will reduce the payment to the 85 percent rate. Reimbursement is made to the PA's employer. It is possible, however, for certain services provided by PAs to be paid at 100 percent of the fee schedule under Medicare's "incident to" or "shared billing" provisions. Both provisions are discussed in detail in later sections.

TYPES OF SERVICES
Services typically reimbursed when performed by a physician are reimbursed when performed by a physician assistant. As allowed by state law, PAs are covered for performing the following: (Note: this list is not all-inclusive.)
- All levels of evaluation and management services (E&M), including levels 4 and 5
- Consultations
- Initial hospital H&Ps
- Mental health services
- All diagnostic tests (ordering and performing)
- First assisting at major surgeries
- Performing minor surgery
- Telemedicine services
- Ordering physical therapy/plan of care
- Signing the certificate of medical necessity for durable medical equipment (DME)

Certain program restricted services, such as routine physicals, are generally not covered under Medicare's fee-for-service program when performed by a physician or a PA. Services such as routine physicals may be covered in rural health clinics or under Medicare HMO plans. Most medically necessary services the PA is authorized to perform by state law will be covered within the Medicare program.

MEDICARE SUPERVISION GUIDELINES
Medicare follows the PA regulations established in each state regarding the degree of supervision required in all practice settings. Under Medicare guidelines, the physician supervisor need not be physically present with the PA when a service is being furnished to a Medicare patient, unless required by state law or in the case of hospitals, by hospital regulations. However, if the physician supervisor (or physician designee) is not physically present with the PA, he or she must be immediately available to the PA for consultation purposes by telephone or other effective, reliable means of communication.

Medicare does not require that physicians cosign PA charts or orders, unless required by state law.

MEDICARE PROVIDER NUMBERS: PIN/UPIN
All PAs who treat or are likely to treat Medicare patients must have their own provider identification number (PIN) and unique provider identification number (UPIN). PINs are used for billing purposes. They identify the person performing the service and, for PAs, also indicate at what percentage the service should be reimbursed (85%). PINs are linked to the employer's tax identification number. So, PAs with multiple employers will have multiple PINs. PAs changing employers must also obtain a new PIN. UPINs are used to identify the person who is ordering diagnostic tests or procedures that are not performed in the office. UPINs are not linked to employers and therefore stay with providers throughout their time within the Medicare program. UPINs are automatically issued after the PIN is issued. UPINs are permanent and do not change when PAs change employers.

To obtain an enrollment application, contact your local Medicare carrier and request the CMS 855I enrollment form.

BILLING MEDICARE IN THE OFFICE OR CLINIC SETTING

Services provided by a PA are reimbursed at 85 percent of the physician fee schedule and should be submitted under the PA's provider number. State law determines supervision and scope of practice. PAs may treat new patients and established patients with new problems and are not required to have the physician physically on-site, unless required by state law or unless the practice is trying to utilize the "incident to" billing provision.

"INCIDENT TO" BILLING

"Incident to" is a Medicare billing provision that allows services provided by PAs in a private office or clinic to be reimbursed at 100 percent of the physician fee schedule. For a practice to bill for medical services provided by PAs under the "incident to" to provision, all the following criteria must be met:

- The physician must personally treat the patient and establish the diagnosis on the patient's visit for that particular medical condition.
- The PA can provide subsequent care for that medical condition.
- The physician must be in the suite of offices when the PA renders follow-up care.

Of course, the physician is responsible for the overall care of the patient and should perform services at a frequency that reflects his or her active and ongoing participation in the management of the patient's course of treatment. There are no national guidelines that determine the frequency of direct physician involvement in the ongoing management of the patient.

"Incident to" is only applicable in a private office or clinic setting. It may not be utilized in nursing facilities, hospitals, or hospital-based or affiliated offices or clinics.

BILLING NON-"INCIDENT TO"

If you cannot meet the guidelines of "incident to" or believe that following "incident to" billing is overly complicated, then virtually any Medicare-covered service may be billed using the PA's PIN with payment at 85 percent of the physician fee schedule. PAs can treat new patients or established patients with new medical problems. In addition, when billing under the PA's PIN, the supervising physician does not have to be on-site when care is provided (unless required by state law).

BILLING MEDICARE IN THE HOSPITAL SETTING

Services provided by the PA in the hospital setting should be billed under the PA's provider number with reimbursement made at 85 percent of the physician fee schedule. State law determines supervision and scope of practice. The physician supervisor need not be physically present with the PA in the hospital when a service is being rendered unless required by state law or hospital regulations.

MEDICARE AND SHARED BILLING IN THE HOSPITAL SETTING

"Incident to" is not an available billing option in the hospital setting. Hospitals can, however, maximize PA reimbursement to 100 percent under Medicare's shared billing provision. PAs and physicians who work for the same employer may share visits made to the same patients on the same day by combining the work of both providers under the physician at 100 percent of the fee schedule. For a hospital visit to be billed under the shared billing provision, the following criteria must be met:

- Both the PA and physician must work for the same employer (e.g., same group practice, same hospital, or PA is employed by a solo physician).
- The regulation applies to E/M services and not procedures or consultations.
- The physician must provide some face-to-face portion of the E/M visit. Simply reviewing or signing the patient's chart is not sufficient.

If the physician does not provide a face-to-face portion of the E/M encounter, then the service is appropriately billed under the PA's PIN with reimbursement at the 85 percent rate.

MEDICARE AND HOSPITAL-EMPLOYED PAs

In the past, Medicare gave hospitals two options for covering services by hospital-employed PAs. Services provided by PAs could be billed under Medicare Part B as a professional service, or the PA's salary could be included in the hospital's cost reports and covered under Medicare Part A.

Because of Medicare's shift to a prospective payment system, the option of including the PA's salary in the hospital's cost reports is no longer an appropriate method of coverage. Some hospitals may not be fully aware of this policy change.

MEDICARE BILLING IN NURSING FACILITIES

Services provided by PAs in nursing facilities should be billed under the PA's provider number with reimbursement at 85 percent of the physician fee schedule. Services should be billed at the physician rate. Medicare will reduce the payment to the 85 percent rate. Although the physician must continually supervise the overall medical care of the nursing home patient, nursing home visits may be delegated to the PA. After the patient's admittance to the facility, Medicare requires that the patient be seen at least once every 30 days for the first 90 days and every 60 days thereafter. The initial comprehensive visit must be made by the physician. After the initial comprehensive visit, the PA and physician may alternate every other required visit. When the PA is performing a nursing home or skilled nursing home visit, Medicare allows PAs to write, sign, and date all progress notes and does not require physician counter-signature unless required by state law.

It is important to be aware of Medicare's specific regulations in **skilled nursing facilities**. Medicare requires that certain medical duties in skilled nursing facilities be performed by a physician. Medicare regulations state that in a skilled nursing facility, a task may not be delegated to a PA when any regulations specify that it must be performed by the physician personally or when delegation to a PA is prohibited by either state law or the policies/regulations of the nursing facility.

In **nursing facilities**, as opposed to skilled nursing facilities, if allowed by state law, PAs may perform services that Medicare regulations state must be performed by the physician. However, if the PA is an employee of that nursing home and is also performing these "physician only" tasks, coverage is not allowed. Medicare coverage is allowed when a PA is an employee of the nursing facility and performing other medically necessary duties that are not designated as "physician only" services.

MEDICAID

Presently, all 50 states cover medical services provided by PAs under their Medicaid fee-for-service or Medicaid managed care programs. The rate of reimbursement, which is generally paid to the PA's employer, is either the same as or slightly lower than that paid to physicians.

PRIVATE INSURANCE

Private health insurance companies do not necessarily follow Medicare's coverage policy rules. As private entities, they are able to establish their own rules and procedures. The potential variation in policy among the various payers makes it imperative that each payer be contacted to determine their specific payment and coverage policies for PAs. Even within the same insurance company, PA coverage policies can change based on the particular plan that an individual or group has selected, the specific type of service being provided, and the part of the country in which the service is delivered.

Most private payers do cover medical and surgical services provided by PAs. Some payers will separately credential and issue provider numbers to PAs. Others ask that services delivered by PAs be billed under the name and provider number of the PA's supervising physician. When a private payer asks for the service to be billed under the name of the supervising physician, it does not necessarily mean that the payer is suggesting that the rules of Medicare's "incident to" billing be utilized. Often payers will defer to supervision requirements as required by state law, even when PA's services are billed under the name and provider number of the supervising physician.

Here are some sample questions you should ask when trying to clarify a company's policies.

- Do you cover medical or surgical first assisting services provided by PAs when working with the supervision of a physician?
- Are PAs credentialed or enrolled?
- Are PAs issued provider numbers? If not, is it acceptable to submit bills under the supervising physician's provider number?
- Can the PA see the patient on the initial office visit?
- Are there any specific supervision requirements? Do you defer to state law?
- Do you defer to state law regarding the services PAs can provide?
- Is coverage also provided in the hospital setting?

Never bill for services provided by a PA under the physician's name and provider number unless you are certain this is approved company policy. It is important to be aware of all company policies and restrictions to ensure proper reimbursement.

MEDICARE POLICY CHART FOR PAs

SETTING	SUPERVISION REQUIREMENT	REIMBURSEMENT RATE	SERVICES
Office / Clinic when physician is not on-site	State Law	85% of physician's fee schedule	All services PA is legally authorized to provide that would have been covered if provided personally by a physician
Office / Clinic when physician is on-site	Physician must be in the suite of offices	100% of physician's fee schedule[1]	Same as above
Home Visit / House Call[2]	State Law	85% of physician's fee schedule	Same as above
Skilled Nursing Facility & Nursing Facility	State Law	85% of physician's fee schedule	Same as above
Hospital	State Law	85% of physician's fee schedule	Same as above
First assisting at surgery in all settings	State Law	85% of physician's first assist fee schedule[3]	Same as above
Federal Rural Health Clinic	State Law	Cost-based reimbursement	Same as above

[1] Using carrier guidelines for "incident to" services.

[2] Not to be confused with home health services.

[3] i.e., 85% x 16% = 13.6% of primary surgeon's fee.

MEDICARE PROVIDER IDENTIFICATION NUMBERS

All PAs who treat or are likely to treat Medicare patients must have their own Provider Identification Numbers (PINs), even if they are in an office or clinic setting where they are primarily utilizing the "incident to" provision. While they may not always use the PIN for billing, the unique provider identification number (UPIN) must be utilized when making referrals or ordering diagnostic tests and procedures.

Just because a PA has a Medicare PIN doesn't mean that it always has to be used for billing purposes. PAs who are in certain specialties, such as pediatrics, where the likelihood of treating a Medicare beneficiary is remote, may choose not to apply.

PINs that are not used in a consecutive 12-month period may become void and must be reactivated.

Contact your local Medicare carrier to request a CMS 855 I provider/supplier general enrollment form. Your Medicare carrier phone number can be obtained from your billing department, the CMS Web site at *www.cms.hhs.gov*, or AAPA. When applying for a PIN, you will need to supply the following:

- the carrier with the name of your employer (either W-2 or 1099 relationship)
- valid state license or temporary license

It will take about 60 days after applying to receive your PIN; if you encounter undue delay, contact AAPA's Government and Professional Affairs reimbursement staff for assistance.

PAS SHOULD APPLY FOR NEW NPI NUMBERS

BY *Michael Powe*

Reprinted from AAPA News, *July 15, 2005*

The Centers for Medicare and Medicaid Services (CMS) announced that, as of May 23, 2005, all health care professionals can apply for a National Provider Identifier (NPI) number. The purpose of the new NPI system is to uniquely identify each health care professional or health care organization that has a need to electronically transmit or receive health care information.

When fully implemented, the 10-digit NPI number will be the one identifying number used by virtually every public and private health insurance plan to recognize health care professionals and health care organizations (e.g., hospitals, nursing facilities, diagnostic testing facilities, etc.). The NPI will replace Medicare's provider identification number (PIN), unique provider identification number (UPIN), and the identification numbers currently in use by private payers.

The Administrative Simplification provisions of the Health Insurance Portability and Accountability Act of 1996 (HIPAA) mandated the use of unique standardized identifiers for all health care professionals, health insurance plans, and health care organizations. The goal of these provisions is to improve the efficiency and effectiveness of the transmission of health care information such as claims data, eligibility inquiries, referrals, and the appropriate communication of other patient medical information. Health care professionals must begin using their NPIs by May 23, 2007. Small health plans have until May 23, 2008.

An application for the NPI number is available on the Web at *https://nppes.cms.hhs.gov*. Medicare, Medicaid, and most private payers will inform health care professionals when NPIs will be officially placed in use for health care transactions.

Section VII

WHAT YOU NEED TO KNOW —
MALPRACTICE
INSURANCE

PROFESSIONAL LIABILITY INSURANCE ESSENTIAL FOR PAs

PAs ARE PROFESSIONALS

When you graduate from PA school and begin practice, you legally become a professional. This means you (and your actions) are judged at higher standards than the general public. Just as any individual can be found liable for injuries or damages suffered in auto accidents, you now can also be found liable for injuries to patients caused in your PA services and performance.

PROFESSIONALS NEED SPECIAL CAREER PROTECTION

This is no minor distinction. Just as you need auto insurance to protect you against damage-recovery lawsuits after an auto accident, you also need insurance to protect you against malpractice lawsuits brought by patients reporting bad-treatment outcomes. Such insurance is usually provided through a professional liability policy, so called because it covers your exposure to liability arising from your profession, including but not limited to, allegations of malpractice. Often, it is just called "malpractice insurance" after the core coverage most third parties are concerned that you have.

YOU NEED PROTECTION FROM DAY ONE

A malpractice incident can happen at any career stage: your first week of practice or the last week before you retire after 30 years. Being new to practice does not lessen your liability risk. Malpractice insurance fees should be viewed as an unavoidable cost of doing business as a PA like paying taxes or dealing with reimbursement forms and procedures.

WHAT YOU DON'T KNOW CAN HURT YOU

In most cases, you will rely on your employer to provide your professional liability insurance, much as you will rely on them to provide your health insurance. Unlike health insurance, you will probably not be asked to contribute to the cost from your paycheck. This will make you even less inclined to question what type of professional liability insurance your employer is providing. But there are two major reasons why you must know about your insurance coverage rather than default to a head-in-the-sand attitude.

HERE TODAY AND GONE TOMORROW...

The Time Element: a malpractice suit can be brought against you after you have seen the patient — often many years later. A neonate you see today can bring a lawsuit 18 years from now on reaching the age of majority. By then, you may be five, six, or more jobs from that initial employment. Your first employer, a local hospital, may have been acquired by another health care system, which merged with another health care system. The original corporate identity of your former employer may no longer exist. Or, your first employer may have gone bankrupt. When you are then sued, to whom do you turn for a defense of the malpractice claim? Your current employer will have no interest in getting involved with a claim from your initial employment. If you have your own professional liability policy, rather than employer-provided coverage, will it go backward to cover that old incident? It's possible, but unlikely. If only you had a copy of the insurance policy that covered you during that first year of employment! You could then contact that insurance company and ask them to respond to the claim on your behalf. Otherwise, you're on your own.

IT'S NOT JUST ABOUT THE MONEY...

Your Reputation: A malpractice suit not only exposes you to financial loss, it also jeopardizes your professional reputation and credentials. For example, as the result of an auto accident, you could lose your driver's license. Similarly, as the result of a malpractice incident, you could lose your license to practice as a PA. You could lose your ability to earn income in spite of the years of training and expense you incurred to become a PA. Even if your license is not revoked or suspended, your ability to work could still be impaired because employers will verify your malpractice history and be reluctant to hire you if you have multiple malpractice incidents or even a single severe incident. It is vital that malpractice suits are vigorously defended. You cannot be a passive participant and just assume your best interests are assured under your employer's insurance. You may be surprised to discover years later that a malpractice case, of which you were blameless, was settled for $1 million with payment allocated to you as a defendant. Under the law, this event was reported to the federal government. The importance of your PA school grade point average fades as you gain actual practice experience, but malpractice settlements stay in a government databank, a part of your "permanent record" forever.

THE TWO SOURCES OF PROFESSIONAL LIABILITY INSURANCE

There are two basic ways to acquire professional liability insurance: your employer puts you on a corporate group policy *or* your employer buys, or reimburses you for, your own individual policy.

Individual Coverage Is Better. For your needs the individual approach is preferred because you control the proof of insurance. Your individual policy serves as separate coverage documentation for you to retain indefinitely letting you avoid reliance on an employer to verify coverage to you, when you need it, possibly many years later after you have moved on to other employment.

Avoid "he said, she said." Because the policy is in your name, the insurer protects only your interests avoiding conflict-of-interest actions likely to arise when serving multiple defendants. For example, suppose a group policy covers both you and your supervising physician and it is established that an error was made. You claim the physician made the error. He claims you did. Can the insurer effectively defend you both?

You have undiluted protection. On a group policy, you may share coverage with other employees. If the amount of coverage (or policy limit) totals $1 million and you share that coverage with other staff, and if a fellow PA is held liable for the $1 million, there is no insurance left. You are unprotected in the event you are also found liable or if there is a future claim.

You can moonlight. The individual policy should cover you on any additional job, whether moonlighting or volunteering. A group policy will only cover you in the scope of your primary employment.

It is portable. Your policy should protect you and move with you from job to job. If you leave your initial employer, your new employer may just reimburse you for maintaining your current policy rather than requiring you to cancel it and move to the group policy. Often, it is actually cheaper for the employer to reimburse your costs than pay additional fees to add you to the group coverage.

Group coverage: Why you can't always get what you want...
In spite of these advantages to you, your employer may just refuse to reimburse you for an individual policy insisting you be covered on the group policy because

It's not win-win. Some previously specified advantages to you of having an individual policy amount to employer disadvantages. For example, you would have your own attorney representing your interests. An employer typically would prefer a single attorney to manage a "global" settlement of any claim. As mentioned, though, this convenience to the employer could ultimately be at your expense if you are held primarily liable.

Not an option for the employer. The employer's insurer may simply not permit an employee to be covered individually. Insurers too do not want to deal with your attorney AND the plaintiff's attorney in negotiating a claim settlement. Also, they sometimes want to retain your coverage premium rather than lose it to another insurer.

SEEKING AN IDEAL INDIVIDUAL POLICY

If you can take the preferred route of an individual policy, asking the following questions can help:

Is the insurer rated "Excellent" or better? An insurance policy is only as good as the assets of the granting insurance company. If the insurer goes out of business, there will be nothing or, at best, pennies-on-the-dollar payment to cover claims. An independent rater of insurer financial strength, A. M. Best & Company, assigns "Excellent," "Very Good," "Good," and other designations to characterize the relative viability of virtually every instance company. Avoid any company lacking A++, A+, A, or A- (Excellent) rating. Lower-rated companies are less likely to exist when you need them. Some companies are not rated at all. This should be taken as even worse than a non-Excellent rating.

Is the policy an occurrence or claims-made policy? If it is claims-made, you need to consider buying tail coverage if you ever terminate the policy and neglect to replace it with similar coverage. You do not have to worry about this with occurrence coverage. But claims-made coverage allows you to maintain a retroactive date which, in effect, covers you backward for

---

Types of Coverage

Occurrence Form: *Insurance that covers medical incidents occurring during the policy period regardless of the date the claim is reported. Upon termination of the policy, coverage still exists if the incident occurred during the policy period. Claims-made form: Insurance that only covers a medical incident that has occurred after the policy's retroactive date and been reported to the insurance company while the policy is in effect. Upon termination of the policy, coverage no longer exists regardless of the date of the incident unless tail coverage has been purchased.*

Tail Coverage (Extended Reporting Endorsement): *Extended Reporting Endorsement attaches to the policy and allows the insured to continue to report incidents that happened during the policy period after the claims-made policy has ended. Tail coverage is bought from the same company that provided the claims-made policy. Extended Reporting Endorsement helps eliminate gaps in the PA's liability insurance coverage.*

patient claims made before the activation of your current policy. The advantage: Even if the insurance company you had way back then is now out of business, your current insurer will cover it. Occurrence lacks this feature. Also, occurrence requires you to retain policy documentation forever. A claim can be brought many years after patient contact. With claims-made, only your current policy is relevant from your policy retroactive date to present.

Is there a "Consent to Settle" provision? Under the terms of an insurance policy, the insurer has not only the duty but also the right to defend and settle claims against you. If the insurer wants to settle for $1 million, it can do so whether you feel you committed malpractice or not. Of course, it does not make sense for the insurer to roll over if you are not at fault, but it is quite possible that the insurer's view of the defensibility of the case and your opinion could clash. That is why most policies now feature "Consent to Settle," requiring that the insurer advise you of a settlement offer before it is finalized. Otherwise, you could find out years later that the $1 million is now on your permanent record, barring you from qualifying for employment at many health care facilities. However, most consent provisions have been watered down over the past few years. The insurer must still obtain your consent, but if you refuse, you will be liable for the difference between the settlement amount and any final verdict. So, you'd better be really sure you're going to win. But use of the consent provision at least provides you the opportunity to influence a final settlement through the consent process.

Is coverage limited to specified employers, work settings, or specialties? The policy should cover you as "Named Insured" without practice restrictions. For example, you may assist in surgery but occasionally work a shift in the ER. There should not be a restriction limiting coverage to your surgical assist duties. If you add a moonlighting job, you should not have to revisit the insurer to add it on to your policy. Note: All insurance policies have exclusions (things the policy will not cover). They are clearly labeled as such in a specific section of the policy called Exclusions. Although reading an insurance policy can be tedious, you really should look these over. Many will be self-evident, i.e., the policy will not cover you for driving an automobile (that requires a different kind of policy). But you may find other restrictions unacceptable, i.e., an exclusion for specific surgical procedures like gastric bypass. If a procedure you perform is excluded, see if your insurer will lift that exclusion.

Is the defense-costs coverage beyond policy limits? Insurers make two basic kinds of payment: indemnity and expense. Indemnity payments go to the injured patient as the result of a settlement or court verdict against you. Expense payments go to the defending law firm that represents you in the suit. Defense costs can often exceed the indemnity payment. Certainly they do if you win in court, as there is no indemnity payment at all. Defense costs can easily go into the six figures and are an important component of your coverage. Some policies limit defense costs by making them part of the policy limits. For example, if the verdict is $500,000 and the defense costs are $500,000, a policy limit of $1 million covers it. If the verdict is $1 million at the same defense costs, you are on the hook for the additional $500,000 since you now exceed policy limits. A preferred policy will not limit defense costs but rather, cover all costs until the policy limit is exhausted by the indemnity payment. Therefore, with the $1 million verdict and $1 million policy limit, the defense costs of $500,000 (or even if it is more) are also covered.

Is there loss-of-income coverage? When you're sued, you likely will devote many hours to testifying at trial and pretrial meetings. If the lawsuit is based on patient contact as part of your current job, your employer will likely not dock you for missing work to comply, but the suit could be based on prior employment elsewhere. It is unlikely your current employer will give carte blanche for that. Loss of income coverage will reimburse you for lost wages (up to the policy limit).

Is there licensure-review coverage? This reimburses you for the cost of legal counsel to represent you at licensure or administrative proceedings to defend your credentials.

Is there coverage for depositions? You may be required to testify in cases where you are not a defendant. However, based on how you answer questions, you may become one. It behooves you to have legal counsel defending your pretrial testimony (called a deposition).

What to Look For in a Group Policy

If your employer insists on your participation in the group policy:

Ask for documentation of coverage. Get a copy of the complete policy if possible. Otherwise, a "Certificate of Insurance" summarizes the terms of coverage. You should get a new one each year, regardless of whether your employer's coverage is occurrence or claims-made. If it is claims-made, you should continue to get a new certificate each year even after you leave that employer unless the employer provides you with evidence that tail coverage was purchased specifically for you. More likely, your tail exposure will be covered by the employer's policy without purchase of tail coverage as long as the employer continuously maintains a policy. However, to verify that the employer has maintained that policy, you must obtain evidence of it annually. Otherwise you will never know if coverage lapsed, in which case your tail coverage stops, and even if the policy is maintained, you will not know who the insurer is should you need to report a claim directly.

Check the insurer's financial rating. Verify that it is A- (Excellent) or better. If it is less, consider out-of-pocket purchase of your own policy, especially if the company is unrated. A "Surplus Lines" or "Non-Admitted" company is all right as long as it has an Excellent rating. If your employer's insurer goes broke, your coverage stops. If your employment agreement included an indemnification from the employer to you, and not just an agreement to obtain insurance, then you may be protected to extent of the employer's assets. However, if a lack of insurance causes the employer to also go broke, you are on your own to the extent of your personal assets. The financial condition of the insurer is critically important. In fact, recheck the insurer's rating every year even if the insurer stays the same from year to year. The rating can change significantly in the space of one year. If your employer's insurance is shaky, you should seriously consider if you want to stay there or at least, get your own policy at your own expense.

For further information, contact:

AAPA Insurance Services
Attn: Gary McCammon
11 South LaSalle Street, Suite 2300
Chicago, IL 60606

312/578-9554 or 877/356-2272

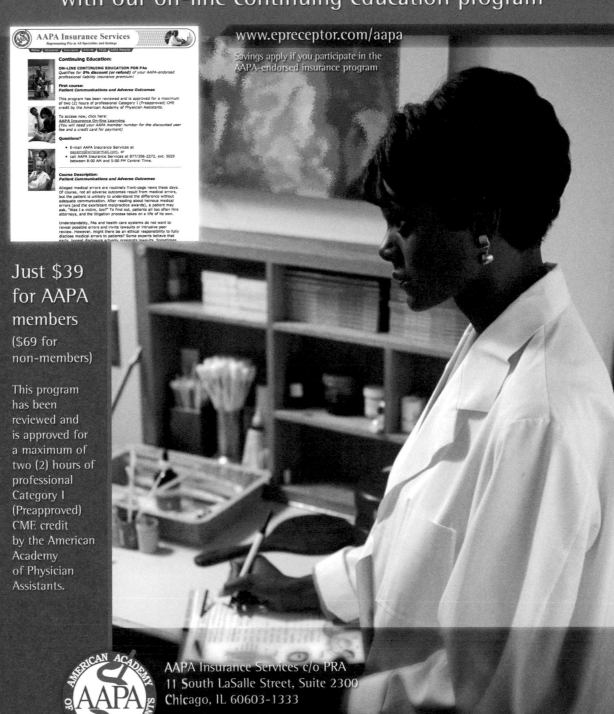
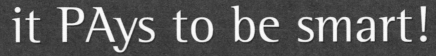

Section VIII

What You Need to Know —
PAs in the Hospital Setting

PAs in Hospital Practice

As a new graduate PA, if you are going to do any work in a hospital, you must obtain hospital privileges first. Your supervising physician has to be a member of the medical staff before you can apply for privileges. Hospitals have some options about setting up a process for privileging PAs, but most likely, you will apply through the medical staff.

The first thing the credentialing staff at the hospital will do is check your basic professional credentials — that is, PA program graduation, state license (unless you are a federal employee), and NCCPA certification. They will also require proof of medical liability insurance coverage, either your own policy or through your employer.

Once you are over that credentials hurdle, they will start looking at the specific privileges you have requested. They will be looking for assurance from your supervising physician and other evidence that you are qualified to perform the privileges requested. They will ask for proof of relevant training or experience and proof of your ability to perform privileges requested. In the case of a new graduate PA, they may accept procedure logs from PA student rotations, letters from supervising physicians during rotations, or letters from your PA program faculty.

The following document is AAPA policy and is primarily intended as a resource for PAs who want to work in hospitals that have never privileged PAs or for hospital medical staffs that are updating obsolete bylaws. It may also help you to understand the process of obtaining hospital privileges.

Guidelines for Amending Medical Staff Bylaws

To provide patient care services in the hospital, physician assistants and their supervising physicians must seek delineation of their clinical privileges. The criteria and process for granting clinical privileges to physician assistants is similar to the process for physicians and should be outlined in the medical staff bylaws.

In most hospitals, the medical staff credentialing process involves simultaneous consideration of applications for medical staff membership and clinical privileges. The following guidelines are intended to assist medical staffs in making appropriate changes to the bylaws that authorize the granting of membership and clinical privileges to physician assistants. They are intended to be a general guide that can be applied and adapted to suit the requirements of individual medical staffs. Where possible, sample language has been included.

Definition of Physician Assistant

Medical staff bylaws usually begin with a section that includes definitions of terms. This section should include a definition of "physician assistant." It should generally conform to the definition used in state law and may reflect the definition used by AAPA (See page 85). In the case of federally employed PAs, the legal definition is found in federal regulations or policies, rather than in state law.

All states require that a physician assistant be a graduate of a PA program accredited by the Accreditation Review Commission on Education for the Physician Assistant (ARC-PA) or one of its predecessor agencies, that they pass the initial exam given by the National Commission on Certification of Physician Assistants (NCCPA), and/or that they be licensed to practice as a physician assistant. Federally employed PAs must meet the first two criteria, but need not be licensed. Some states and employers require current NCCPA certification.

The following definition serves as an example:
A physician assistant (PA) is an individual who is a graduate of a physician assistant program approved by the Accreditation Review Commission on Education for the Physician Assistant (ARC-PA) or one of its predecessor agencies, and/or has been certified by the National Commission on Certification of Physician Assistants (NCCPA). The individual meets the necessary legal requirements for licensure to practice medicine with physician supervision.

PAs on the Medical Staff

Physician assistants should be members of the medical staff. Physician assistants are providers of physician services. They exercise a high level of decision making and autonomy in providing patient care, although they practice as supervised members of physician-directed teams. Membership on the medical staff enables providers to diagnose illness and perform other functions in the hospital. It allows providers a voice in developing and implementing hospital and medical staff policies and ensures participation in programs to review the quality and appropriateness of patient care. It is important that PAs participate in the system in which medical care policies are made and communicated.

Sometimes medical staff attorneys mistakenly believe that standards from the Joint Commission on Accreditation of Health Care Organizations (JCAHO) prohibit physician assistant membership on the medical staff. The standards state that the medical staff includes physicians and may include other licensed independent practitioners. According to JCAHO correspondence with AAPA, this is not meant to be exclusive language, and medical staffs may choose to include PAs as

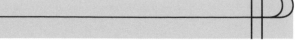

members. The Medicare Conditions of Participation for Hospitals clearly state that in addition to M.D. and D.O. members, the medical staff "may also be composed of other practitioners appointed by the governing body." State law should be consulted; sometimes the makeup of medical staff membership is dictated there.

Physician assistants are providers of medical care and should not be categorized under nursing. Similarly, categorization under allied health is inappropriate. AAPA is not alone in this viewpoint. The National Commission on Allied Health, convened by an act of Congress in 1992, defined an allied health professional as "a health professional (other than a registered nurse or physician assistant) who has received a certificate, an associate degree, a bachelor's degree, a master's degree, a doctoral degree, or post-baccalaureate training in a science related to health care … etc." The federal Bureau of Health Professions uses this same definition, excluding PAs from the allied health professions and classifying them as medical care providers.

Medical staff membership language might state:
Membership on the medical staff shall be extended to physicians, dentists, podiatrists, physician assistants, and clinical psychologists who continuously meet the qualifications, standards, and requirements set forth in these bylaws and who are appointed by the hospital Board of Directors.

Credentialing Physician Assistants

Medical staff bylaws specify professional criteria for medical staff membership and clinical privileges. JCAHO specifies four core criteria that should be met when credentialing licensed independent practitioners, including current licensure, relevant training or experience, current competence (defined as letters from authoritative sources attesting to the applicant's scope and level of performance), and the ability to perform privileges requested. This serves as a reasonable guideline. As applied to physician assistants, these criteria might include evidence of current state licensure; relevant training and/or experience; national certification; letters from previous employers, supervising physicians, or PA programs attesting to scope and level of performance; attestation as to physical and mental health status; evidence of adequate professional liability insurance, information on any past or pending professional liability or disciplinary actions, and a supervising physician (M.D. or D.O.) who is a member of the medical staff.

Physician Assistant Privileges

The medical staff bylaws should require each PA to have clinical privileges and proper physician supervision, regardless of whether the PA is an employee of a practice or of the hospital. Medical staff membership should not be a requirement for granting of clinical privileges. This is in accordance with JCAHO standards and the Medicare Conditions of Participation for Hospitals.

The medical staff bylaws should stipulate that all clinical privileges granted to a physician assistant should be consistent with all applicable state and federal laws and regulations and that a physician assistant may provide medical and surgical services as delegated by a supervising physician. Typically, privileges for a physician assistant are delineated using a form and process identical to or very similar to that used for their supervising physician. Because PAs provide physician services, the physician form and privileging system is a useful template for developing a system of granting PA privileges.

The process for granting clinical privileges is usually discussed in four places in the bylaws: the article concerned with clinical privileges, the article describing the structure of the credentials committee, the article describing the duties of department chairs, and the article describing hearing procedures. The process of granting clinical privileges may vary considerably from one hospital to another, but generally the process should: (1) be completed in a timely fashion; (2) if they exist, department chairs should make specific recommendations for clinical privileges; (3) an appeal mechanism for adverse decisions should exist; and (4) the governing board should have ultimate authority to grant clinical privileges. An application for renewal of clinical privileges should be processed in essentially the same manner as that for granting initial privileges.

The criteria for delineating clinical privileges should be specified in the bylaws. They are usually the same as those used for credentialing: evidence of current state licensure, relevant training and experience, national certification, letters from authoritative sources attesting to the individual's ability to perform certain privileges, attestation as to physical and mental health status, evidence of adequate liability insurance, and information on any past or pending professional liability or disciplinary actions. Privilege determinations — at reappointment or other interim times — might also include observed clinical performance, quality improvement data, and other documented results of quality improvement activities required by the hospital and medical staff.

Other requirements of physician members of the medical staff also may apply to PAs. For instance, if a department chair approves physician privilege requests before they are submitted to the medical staff credentials committee, the same should apply to PAs. If demonstrated, documented competency is required for physicians requesting new privileges, the same should be required of PAs.

When credentialing a PA, a query should be made to the National Practitioner Data Bank (NPDB) regarding his or her medical liability history. Entities that make malpractice payments on behalf of PAs must report that information to the NPDB. Employers and regulators are not required to report adverse professional review actions taken against PAs to the NPDB. As a result, that information in the NPDB is incomplete. Queries about licensure actions taken against PAs can be made to the Federation of State Medical Boards (FSMB). Although all state licensing boards are encouraged to report disciplinary actions to the FSMB, it is impossible to ascertain whether all actions are reported, so it is important that hospitals also query individual licensing boards.

DURATION AND RENEWAL OF APPOINTMENTS

Duration of appointments and privileges should be the same for physicians and physician assistants. The renewal process also should be similar.

Due Process

The bylaws should give the physician assistant the right to request the initiation of due process procedures when actions taken by the medical staff or the governing board adversely affect his or her clinical privileges. Hospital accreditation standards from JCAHO specifically state that medical staffs must establish a fair hearing and appeals process for addressing adverse decisions made against medical staff members and others holding clinical privileges. The process should include PA peer reviewers.

Corrective Action

The criteria and process for disciplining physician assistants should be spelled out in the bylaws. The process should involve PA peers and conform to the process applied to physician members of the medical staff.

AAPA AND AMA PARTNER TO OFFER STATE-OF-THE-ART PA CREDENTIAL VERIFICATION SERVICE

By Christopher Doscher

Reprinted from AAPA News, October 15, 2005

AAPA received more than 15,000 requests for PA credentialing information in the less than two years since it partnered with the American Medical Association (AMA) to add verification of PA credentials to the AMA's well-known Physician Profile Service.

The service, launched in November 2003, allows professionals who verify credentials applications for hospitals or managed care organizations to verify PA certification and current status of certification, the program from which the PA graduated and graduation date, current and historical state licensure information, and AAPA membership status.

The service eliminates the need for credentialing professionals to contact individual PA programs and the National Commission on Certification of Physician Assistants to verify a PA's credentials application, saving hours of work. The PA profile service is available at a cost of $16 per profile at *https://profiles.ama-assn.org/amaprofiles*.

Hospitals are required to perform primary source verification on data submitted by every clinician that they credential or recredential. The AMA's PA profile service provides such information for both initial credentialing and the biannual recredentialing.

In January 2004, the Joint Commission on Accreditation of Healthcare Organizations began requiring hospitals to credential PAs through the medical staff or an equivalent process, making the PA profile service an even more valuable time-saving tool.

AAPA provides the PA data for the profiling service, but the service itself is operated by the AMA, which handles the requests for information. PAs do not have to take any action or provide any information to be included in the primary source data available through the service. However, PAs should verify the accuracy of information about them, particularly date of birth, by reviewing their record in AAPA's on-line member directory at *https://members.aapa.org* or by calling AAPA CME and Member Services at 703/836-2272, ext. 3350.

Quality Assurance

The bylaws should provide for effective mechanisms to carry out quality assurance responsibilities with respect to physician assistants. These mechanisms should include regular monitoring and evaluation by the supervising physician. Peer review of PA practice should be conducted by peers — ideally other physician assistants in the same area of clinical specialty. If the staff does not include other PAs in the same specialty, PA peers from outside the hospital should be called in.

Continuing Medical Education

The medical staff bylaws should require participation by physician assistants in continuing medical education that relates, at least in part, to their regular practice and to their clinical privileges.

Committees

Bylaws should allow physician assistant membership on medical staff committees.

Discrimination

The fundamental criteria for medical staff membership or clinical privileges should be directly related to the delivery of quality medical care, professional ability and judgment, and community need. Medical staff membership or particular clinical privileges should not be denied on the basis of gender, color, creed, race, religion, age, ethnic or national origin, political beliefs, disability, socioeconomic status, or sexual orientation.

PARTICIPATION IN DISASTER AND EMERGENCY CARE

The bylaws should include language enabling physician assistants to provide care during emergency or disaster situations. The bylaws should state that the chief executive or his or her designee may grant temporary clinical privileges when appropriate and that emergency privileges may be granted when the hospital's emergency management plan has been activated. The hospital's emergency preparedness plan should include physician assistants in its identification of care providers authorized to respond in emergency or disaster situations.

Bylaws language might state:

In case of an emergency, any member of the medical staff, house staff, and any licensed health practitioner, limited only by the qualifications of their license and regardless of service or staff status, shall be permitted to render emergency care. They will be expected to do everything possible to save the life of a patient, utilizing all resources of the hospital as necessary, including the calling of any consultations necessary or desirable. Any physician assistant acting in an emergency or disaster situation shall be exempt from the hospital's usual requirements of physician supervision to the extent allowed by state law in disaster or emergency situations. Any physician who supervises a physician assistant providing medical care in response to such an emergency or declared disaster does not have to meet the requirements set forth in these bylaws for a supervising physician.

Policy Brief: Guidelines for Amending Hospital Staff Bylaws
Adopted 1987; Amended 1993 and 2003

Section IX

What You Need to Know —
Prescribing & Dispensing

OVERVIEW: PRESCRIBING AND DISPENSING

The legal authority for PAs to sign prescriptions has existed in certain states since the 1970s. In the past few years, the number of states recognizing the value of PA prescribing has greatly expanded. Forty-eight states plus the District of Columbia and Guam have passed laws or regulations allowing physicians to delegate their prescriptive authority to PAs. Other states are in the process of changing laws or regulations or are expected to do so in the near future. Federally employed PAs also have been granted prescriptive privileges by most agencies.

A PA's prescriptive authority is always dependent on the delegation of this function by the PA's supervising physician(s).

The laws and regulations for PA prescribing vary by state. They are administered by medical or PA licensing boards, rarely by pharmacy boards. In general, PAs are authorized to sign prescriptions with their names, and prescription blanks are required to bear the name of the PA and the supervising physician. A physician cosignature is not required.

TYPES OF DRUGS

When PAs have prescriptive privileges, it means that, at a minimum, they can sign prescriptions for legend drugs without obtaining a physician cosignature. In 44 states, PAs may also prescribe controlled substances. Twenty-nine states permit PAs to prescribe drugs in Schedules II through V (occasionally with a limitation on the supply of Schedule II drugs or location for Schedule II prescribing); 14 others allow PAs to prescribe drugs in Schedules III through V.

A few state medical boards have developed formularies, or lists of drug categories, to guide prescribing. Some states had formularies in place, then decided they were unnecessary or cumbersome, given that PAs practice in all medical specialties and settings.

DEA REGISTRATION

The federal Drug Enforcement Administration (DEA) established a registration category in 1993 for "midlevel practitioners" (defined as PAs, nurse midwives, nurse practitioners, optometrists, and others), authorized by states to prescribe controlled substances. At the same time, the DEA kept on the books an exemption from registration for those individuals who are agents or employees of authorized and registered prescribers.

In 1997, however, the DEA made it quite clear that PAs who prescribe controlled substances must obtain registration numbers. All state laws or regulations now reflect the DEA's requirement that PAs prescribing controlled substances must register with the DEA.

National surveys reveal that PA prescribing patterns are very similar to those of physicians. In 2005, PAs were responsible for more than 221 million patient visits and wrote prescriptions for 278 million pharmaceutical products.

Very few disciplinary actions against PAs for misuse or abuse of prescriptive privileges can be identified. Likewise, there is no record of significantly increased liability or malpractice claims due to PA prescribing. Professional liability insurers do not increase premiums when PAs are granted authority to prescribe.

DRUG DISPENSING

Approximately 28 jurisdictions allow physicians to delegate dispensing privileges to PAs. Depending on the state, dispensing may be restricted to certain kinds of health care facilities or geographic locations; the quantity of drugs dispensed may also be limited.

Samples

The distribution of pharmaceutical product samples to health care providers was once a largely unregulated activity. When the U.S. Congress uncovered evidence of drug diversion and resale, adulterated and misbranded samples, and the importation of foreign counterfeit drugs, it moved to prevent such abuses. In 1987, Congress enacted the Prescription Drug Marketing Act (PDMA) (Public Law 100-293). Pharmaceutical manufacturers face severe criminal and financial penalties for violating this law, which sets storage, handling, and accounting requirements for drug samples; bans the reimportation of prescription drugs; and prohibits certain wholesale drug distribution practices.

Through the efforts of AAPA, the law contains language allowing individuals "licensed or otherwise authorized by the state to prescribe" to request and sign for drug samples. A letter to AAPA from the Food and Drug Administration (FDA) states that affiliated practitioners (e.g., physician assistants) who are licensed by a state and who have been granted either dependent or independent prescriptive authority are not prohibited, under the PDMA, from requesting and signing for prescription drug samples.

When writing the PDMA, it appears Congress and the FDA envisioned a two-step process for distribution of samples: a request form signed by a prescriber and a receipt form signed by a responsible person on delivery of the product, whether by mail, by common carrier, or by a company representative. If samples were distributed in this fashion, PAs in any state could be the designated recipients because individuals without prescriptive authority can receive samples. However, for record-keeping purposes, pharmaceutical companies have combined the request and receipt into one form. For practical purposes, this means that only PAs with prescriptive privileges may request (i.e., sign for) samples.

Some state legislatures and licensing boards have adopted language describing how PA sampling should be handled. The authority of PAs to request, sign for, and distribute sample medications to patients may match, but not exceed, their prescriptive privileges (that is, samples of controlled substances may be requested or distributed by PAs only if they are allowed to prescribe such drugs).

AAPA encourages all state PA associations to seek modification of their laws or regulations so it is clear that PAs may request, receive, and sign for professional samples and may distribute or supply samples to their patients. Model language has been developed that makes a clear distinction between drug dispensing and distribution of samples. It also explicitly identifies each step in the process of requesting, signing, and distributing samples to patients so that there is no confusion about what PAs are authorized to do.

REFERENCE TO THE CONTROLLED SUBSTANCES ACT OF 1970

The Drug Enforcement Administration's authority to regulate pharmaceutical controlled substances is derived from the Controlled Substances Act (CSA) [21 U.S.C. §§ 801-971]. The CSA mandates that the DEA prevent, detect, and investigate the diversion of legally manufactured controlled substances while, at the same time, ensuring that there are adequate supplies to meet the legitimate medical needs in the United States.

To enable the DEA to achieve these goals, the CSA established five schedules into which controlled substances are separated according to their approved medical use and abuse potential. Schedule I controlled substances are those with a very high potential for abuse and that are deemed not to have legitimate medical uses. Schedule II substances are approved for medical use and also have a very high abuse potential. Schedules III, IV, and V include controlled substances that have all been approved for medical use and have diminishing potential for abuse.

The DEA's schedules for controlled substances change as new medications are developed and the abuse potential of existing medications is re-evaluated. Current information on medications and their schedule designation can be found on the DEA's Web site, *www.deadiversion.usdoj.gov/schedules/schedules/htm.*

The schedules are as follows:

Schedule I Substances
The drugs in this schedule have a high abuse potential and no accepted medical use in the United States. They include heroin, LSD, and mescaline.

Schedule II Substances
The drugs in this schedule have a high abuse potential with severe psychic or physical dependence liability. Schedule II controlled substances consist of certain narcotics, stimulants, and depressants. Examples are hydromorphone (Dilaudid®), meperidine (Demerol®), methylphenidate (Ritalin®), methadone, fentanyl, amphetamine, methamphetamine, morphine, pentobarbital, secobarbital, and oxycodone.

Schedule III Substances
Substances in this schedule have an abuse potential less than those in Schedules I and II and include compounds containing limited quantities of certain narcotic and non-narcotic drugs. Their abuse may lead to moderate or low physical dependence or high psychological dependence. Examples are codeine (Tylenol® with Codeine), hydrocodone combination products, butalbital, pentobarbital combination products, and dihydrotestosterone.

Schedule IV Substances
Substances in this schedule have an abuse potential less than those listed in Schedule III, which may lead only to limited physical dependence or psychological dependence. Schedule IV drugs include butorphanol (Stadol®), chloral hydrate, diazepam, flurazepam, midazolam (Versed®), pemoline (Cylert®), phenobarbitol, sibutramine (Meridia®), zaleplon (Sonata®), zolpidem (Ambien®), dextropropoxyphene dosage forms, and pentazocine (Talwin-NX®).

Schedule V Substances
These substances have an abuse potential less than those listed in Schedule IV and consist primarily of preparations containing limited quantities of certain narcotic and stimulant drugs generally for antitussive, antidiarrheal, and analgesic purposes.

WHERE PHYSICIAN ASSISTANTS ARE AUTHORIZED TO PRESCRIBE

Jurisdiction	Rx Status	Restrictions	Controlled Substances
Alabama	Rx	Formulary	
Alaska	Rx		Sch. III-V
Arizona	Rx		Sch. II-III limited to 14-day supply with board prescribing certification (72-hours without); Sch. IV-V, not more than 5 times in 6-month period per patient
Arkansas	Rx		Sch. III-V
California	Rx	PAs may write "drug orders" which, for the purposes of DEA registration, meet the federal definition of a prescription	Sch. II-V
Colorado	Rx		Sch. II-V
Connecticut	Rx		Sch. II-V
Delaware	Rx		Sch. II-V
District of Columbia	Rx		
Florida	Rx	Formulary of prohibited drugs	
Georgia	Rx	Formulary	Sch. III-V
Guam	Rx		Sch. III-V
Hawaii	Rx		Sch. III-V
Idaho	Rx		Sch. II-V
Illinois	Rx		Sch. III-V
Indiana			
Iowa	Rx		Sch. III-V; Sch. II (except stimulants and depressants)
Kansas	Rx		Sch. II-V
Kentucky	Rx		
Louisiana	Rx		Sch. III-V
Maine	Rx		Sch. III-V (Board may approve Sch. II for individual PAs)
Maryland	Rx		Sch. II-V
Massachusetts	Rx		Sch. II-V
Michigan	Rx		Sch. III-V; Sch. II (7-day supply) as discharge meds
Minnesota	Rx	Formulary	Sch. II-V
Mississippi	Rx		Sch. II-V
Missouri	Rx		
Montana	Rx		Sch. II-V (Sch. II limited to 34-day supply)
Nebraska	Rx		Sch. II-V
Nevada	Rx		Sch. II-V
New Hampshire	Rx		Sch. II-V
New Jersey	Rx		Sch. II-V (certain conditions apply)
New Mexico	Rx	Formulary	Sch. II-V
New York	Rx		Sch. III-V
North Carolina	Rx		Sch. II-V (Sch. II-III limited to 30-day supply)
North Dakota	Rx		Sch. III-V
Ohio			
Oklahoma	Rx	Formulary	Sch. III-V
Oregon	Rx		Sch. II-V
Pennsylvania	Rx	Formulary	Sch. III-V. Limited to 30-day supply unless for chronic condition
Rhode Island	Rx		Sch. II-V
South Carolina	Rx	Formulary	Sch. V
South Dakota	Rx		Sch. II-V (Sch. II limited to 48-hour supply)
Tennessee	Rx		Sch. II-V
Texas	Rx	In specified practice sites	Sch. III-V (limited to 30-day supply)
Utah	Rx		Sch. II-V
Vermont	Rx	Formulary	Sch. II-V
Virginia	Rx		Sch. III-V
Washington	Rx		Sch. II-V
West Virginia	Rx	Formulary	Sch. III-V (Sch. III limited to 72-hour supply)
Wisconsin	Rx		Sch. II-V
Wyoming	Rx		Sch. II-V

DEA Registration: The Drug Enforcement Administration (DEA) has a registration category specifically for physician assistants and other so-called "midlevel practitioners" authorized by state law or regulation to prescribe controlled substances. For more information or to obtain a registration application, contact the DEA Registration Unit at 800/882-9539.

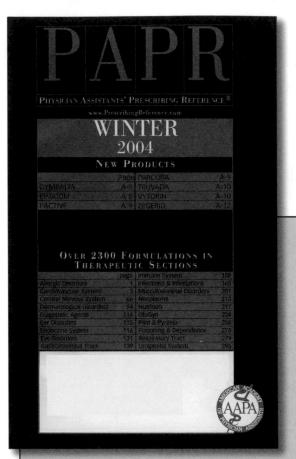

Section X

Your Professional
&
Personal Growth

BE A LEADER

The PA profession is built on individuals working to promote PAs, the profession, and the accomplishments of PAs, and thereby helping PAs continue to gain recognition and status.

As a practicing PA, you will want to get involved with your profession on both the personal and professional levels so that you can take part in helping the profession evolve to the next level.

For personal growth, you might want to work to strengthen your own leadership abilities, find your balance between work and life, reach out to your community, and promote the PA profession. One instrument that AAPA offers for members is the Leadership Toolbox, designed to help you assess your leadership abilities and work to enhance them with self-paced resources derived from a list of core competencies related to leadership.

In addition to personal growth, you will want to consider how you can advance yourself professionally and this might include getting involved as a leader in the profession. AAPA offers you many opportunities to do this, from being a leader of the national organization to helping govern a constituent organization.

Even if you decide not to lead an organization, get involved and help them promote and advance the PA profession, work to strengthen PAs' ties within the community and the organization, and continue to develop yourself professionally and personally.

AAPA PROFESSIONAL & PERSONAL DEVELOPMENT TOOLBOX

AAPA offers a Professional and Personal Development Toolbox for its members. The toolbox, available on the Academy's Web site at *www.aapa.org/toolbox*, contains resources, created from leadership's core competencies, to help you improve and enhance your skills, knowledge, and abilities, which will positively impact your personal life and your PA career.

The toolbox was developed by the AAPA Leadership Advisory Commission (LAC) in 2003-2004. In 2005, LAC's successor, the Leadership & Professional Development Council, assumed management of the toolbox.

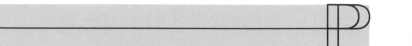

YOUR PROFESSIONAL ASSOCIATIONS

AMERICAN ACADEMY OF PHYSICIAN ASSISTANTS

The American Academy of Physician Assistants, established in April 1968, is the national voice for physician assistants in all medical and surgical specialties. Its early membership consisted of the first graduates of the Duke University PA Program. In 1973, 300 members strong, a joint national office for AAPA and the Association of Physician Assistant Programs (APAP) was opened in Washington, D.C., with an executive director and two support staff. Today, there are nearly 40,000 members representing every state and territory and a national office located in Alexandria, Virginia.

Physician assistants who are graduates of PA educational programs accredited by the Accreditation Review Commission on Education for the Physician Assistant (ARC-PA) or one of its predecessor agencies and those who are certified by the National Commission on Certification of Physician Assistants (NCCPA) are eligible for membership in AAPA. There are also membership categories for students not yet in the PA training phase of their programs, physicians, PAs who have left the profession but wish to support it, other health professionals, and service providers.

Mission and Vision

The Academy's mission, as determined by the House of Delegates, is to promote quality, cost-effective, and accessible health care and to promote the professional and personal development of physician assistants. The vision of the organization is that physician assistants will be worldwide leaders vital to providing and improving the medical care of all people.

Governance of the Academy

The AAPA House of Delegates, the policy-making body of the Academy, meets annually. The House of Delegates is comprised of representatives from chartered constituent chapters, officially recognized specialty PA organizations, the Student Academy of the American Academy of Physician Assistants (SAAAPA), the Physician Assistant Education Association (PAEA), the Caucus Congress, and the immediate past and current House Officers. House delegates elect three officers: Speaker of the House, first vice speaker, and second vice speaker. These three officers serve on the AAPA Board of Directors, along with the president, president elect, secretary, treasurer, immediate past president, four directors at large, and a student representative (SAAAPA immediate past president).

Constituent Organization Structure

The Academy has a federated structure of 57 chartered constituent chapters representing the interests of physician assistants in 50 states, the District of Columbia, Guam, the Air Force, Navy, Army, Public Health Service, and Department of Veterans Affairs. In addition, AAPA officially recognizes specialty organizations, caucuses, and special interest groups. The list of constituent organizations is available on the AAPA Web site, *www.aapa.org*. Other AAPA organizations are the Physician Assistant Foundation, the philanthropic arm of the Academy; SAAAPA, which includes individual student societies from physician assistant programs; and the AAPA Political Action Committee, which supports federal candidates friendly to the PA profession.

Liaisons and Representatives

AAPA leaders are the recognized spokespersons for the PA profession before various national bodies. Paralleling the close working relationship between PAs and physicians, AAPA has developed liaisons with various medical and health care organizations, including the American Medical Association, American College of Surgeons, and the American Academy of Family Physicians.

PHYSICIAN ASSISTANT EDUCATION ASSOCIATION

The Physician Assistant Education Association (PAEA), formerly the Association of Physician Assistant Programs, is the national organization that represents the more than 130 accredited physician assistant programs in the United States accredited by the Accreditation Review Commission on Education for the Physician Assistant (ARC-PA).

The association's mission is to "pursue excellence, foster faculty development, advance the body of knowledge that defines quality education and patient-centered care, and promote diversity in all aspects of physician assistant education."

PAEA's services to its members include a variety of educational programs developed by its Faculty Development Institute, two annual meetings, a peer-reviewed quarterly journal, a directory of faculty and staff, and a research grants program. The association also runs the Central Application Service for Physician Assistants (CASPA), which allows applicants to PA programs to apply to multiple programs through one application and reduces the administrative burden for PA programs, and publishes on-line the Physician Assistant Programs Directory, which helps applicants choose which programs to apply to.

The association's two self-assessment exams have become invaluable study tools for the profession in recent years. PACKRAT, for students preparing for certification, has been revised into an electronic format, e-PACKRAT; the PA GRAD-RAT, designed for graduate PAs preparing for recertification, has been incorporated into the *Comprehensive Review for the Certification and Recertification Examinations for Physician Assistants*.

The association has shared office space with and been managed under contract by the AAPA since shortly after its founding in 1973. In November 2005, the membership voted to change the association's name, taking advantage of a planned move to independent management and to new office space in spring 2006.

Physician Assistant Foundation

The Physician Assistant Foundation serves as the philanthropic arm of AAPA. Founded in 1980, the PA Foundation invests in the future of the physician assistant profession by providing funding for scholarships, service projects, and education programs, as well as advocating and assisting PA involvement in a wide variety of community-based activities.

Structured as a 501(c)(3) organization and governed by a Board of Trustees, the PA Foundation has grown dramatically in recent years and now sponsors several initiatives, including the following:

Innovations in Health Care: The AAPA/PA Foundation/ Pfizer Recognition Program

Sponsored by AAPA, the PA Foundation, and Pfizer Inc, this program recognizes unique innovations in clinical practices and in PA educational programs. Annually, awards in the amount of $5,000 or $3,500 are presented to the physician assistant's practice or an academic institution to support further development and/or implementation of the practice or curriculum. Applications may be downloaded at *www.aapa.org/paf/ innovations-form.pdf.*

Annual Scholarship Program

Since 1989, this program has awarded more than $1 million to PA students across the country. Scholarships in the amount of $2,000 are awarded on the basis of financial need, academic achievement, extracurricular activities, and future goals as a PA. The deadline for 2005-2006 is February 1, 2006. Applications may be downloaded at *www.aapa.org/paf/app-scholarship.html.*

Breitman-Dorn Endowed Research Fellowship

The Breitman-Dorn Endowed Research Fellowship, established in May 1998, encourages a commitment to conduct research in and on the PA profession and provides financial assistance to doctoral candidates who are making a contribution to research on the influence of PAs in medical care. This application and requirements for this $3,000 award may be downloaded at *www.aapa.org/paf/bdfgapp.pdf.*

Community-based Projects Grants: People Helping People

This program, started in 1998 by the PA Foundation, provides seed money for PAs and PA students launching innovative local community programs to improve health and human conditions. Awards of up to $2,500 are granted for community-based initiatives that focus on service, education, and/or research. You may download this application at *www.aapa. org/paf/pafproposal.pdf.* Deadlines for applications are January 1, April 1, July 1, and October 1.

Constituent Organization Matching Grant Program

The purpose of the matching grant program is to provide supplemental funds for awards. Through this program, the PA Foundation will match 85 percent of the funds from a constituent organization or a PA program up to a maximum of $2,500. You may download this application at *www.aapa. org/paf/02PAFmatch-grant-prog-app.pdf.*

Host City Prevention Campaign

The Host City Prevention Campaign (HCPC) is accomplished through the efforts of four PA organizations: AAPA, the PA Foundation, the PA Education Association, and the Student Academy of AAPA. The HCPC project for 2005-2006 is working to eliminate health disparities. More information can be downloaded at *www.aapa.org/paf/hcpc.html.*

Gateways

Gateways is a national PA student leadership program that enables students to succeed in future leadership roles as volunteers within AAPA and as health care providers in their own communities. The program provides skill development and information to help students enhance their leadership abilities, along with opportunities to practice leadership through a special project. The program is in collaboration with the Physician Assistant Education Association and SAAAPA, and with support from Bristol-Myers Squibb Company. The 2006 program will take place at the AAPA's 34th Annual PA Conference in San Francisco. The Gateways application may be downloaded at *www.aapa.org/paf/pafprog.html#gate.*

Healthy Neighborhoods Grant Program

The Healthy Neighborhoods grant initiative provides funding to support, maintain, and expand existing successful projects. This program supports projects that focus on community-based initiatives through service, education, or research. The deadlines for applications are April 1 and November 1. The Healthy Neighborhoods application may be downloaded at *www.aapa.org/paf/pafhngi.pdf.*

Global Outreach Program

The Global Outreach humanitarian assistance program provides grants to support organizations or individuals that work to improve the quality of life in underserved areas of the United States or in developing countries by creating sustainable development in the areas of health care or health education. The deadlines for applications are April 1 and November 1. The Global Outreach application may be downloaded at *www.aapa.org/paf/pafgophag.pdf.*

NATIONAL COMMISSION ON CERTIFICATION OF PHYSICIAN ASSISTANTS

The National Commission on Certification of Physician Assistants (NCCPA) is the only national credentialing organization for physician assistants in the United States. Established as a not-for-profit organization in 1975, NCCPA is dedicated to assuring the public that certified physician assistants meet established standards of knowledge and clinical skills throughout their careers. All 50 states, the District of Columbia, and the U.S. territories rely on NCCPA certification criteria for initial licensure or regulation of physician assistants.

The PA-C designation is a mark of professional accomplishment that is widely recognized within the medical professions and beyond. To attain the designation, PAs must pass NCCPA's Physician Assistant National Certifying Examination (PANCE). Administered to graduates of accredited PA programs, PANCE is a multiple-choice test that assesses entry-level medical and surgical knowledge. After passing PANCE, PAs are issued a certificate entitling them to use the PA-C designation.

To maintain NCCPA certification and to retain the right to use the designation, PAs must follow a process that involves documentation of continuing medical education (CME) credits, submission of reregistration materials and — after six years — successful completion of a recertification exam. All NCCPA exams are developed in conjunction with the National Board of Medical Examiners with the assistance of physicians and physician assistants who are in clinical or academic practice in a variety of practice settings and specialties.

ASSOCIATION OF POSTGRADUATE PA PROGRAMS

The goals of the Association of Postgraduate Physician Assistant Programs (APPAP) include the following:

- Assisting in the development and organization of post-graduate educational curricula and programs for PAs
- Assisting in defining the role of the PA (with emphasis on the specialties)
- Assisting in the development of evaluation methodologies for postgraduate educational curricula and programs

Serving as an information center to PAs, programs training PAs at the entry level, other medical and health care disciplines, and the public with respect to postgraduate educational programs for PAs. All member programs of APPAP are postgraduate PA programs that offer structured curricula, including didactic and clinical components, to train NCCPA-eligible or certified PAs for a defined period of time (usually 12 months) in a medical specialty. APPAP member programs follow several models, including fellowships, master's degree programs, and residencies. All APPAP member programs must award a certificate or degree or provide graduate academic credit.

Section XI

Your Academy Is Here to Help

AAPA AND YOU

As you gear up for an important transition in your life — the move from PA student to clinically practicing PA — you can rely on your professional association to assist you along the way. As the only national association representing physician assistants in every specialty and practice setting, the American Academy of Physician Assistants (AAPA) has developed a comprehensive mix of professional and personal development services designed to assist you with each stage of your career. More than 38,000 practicing PAs and PA students nationwide have found their professional strength and voice in their AAPA membership.

If you've been involved with AAPA as a student member, you already know about the association and some of our membership benefits and services. If you haven't been a member, you are invited to take a look at the many valuable services and resources that are available exclusively to AAPA members. We're confident that you'll find membership in your professional organization to be a valuable supplement to your PA education.

■ FREQUENTLY ASKED QUESTIONS

Q. Where can I find my AAPA membership ID number?

A. Your membership ID number is imprinted on your AAPA membership card. You may also contact AAPA Member & CME Services via e-mail at *aapa@aapa.org* to request it or you can call 703/836-2272, ext. 3350.

Q. I just graduated. When should I convert my student membership to fellow membership?

A. If you graduate during your membership year, you may opt to keep your student membership until your membership renewal date. Your membership will automatically be upgraded to a fellow (graduate) status and you will be sent a renewal notice approximately three months before expiration of your student membership.

You may also choose to upgrade your student membership to fellow membership directly after graduation. Many students choose this option to get a head start on earning required CME credits for certification maintenance. If you choose to upgrade your membership to fellow with time remaining in your student membership, you will receive prorated credit roward your fellow membership. For example:

Jane graduates in August 2006
Jane's student membership expires February 2007 (5 months remaining in membership)
Jane upgrades her student membership to fellow in September 2006
Jane's new fellow membership expires in September 2007

To easily upgrade your membership, simply e-mail Member & CME Services at *aapa@aapa.org* or call 703/836-2272, ext. 3350.

Q. How do I upgrade my student membership to fellow membership?

A. You can wait until you receive your renewal notice, approximately three months prior to your membership expiration, or you can simply contact Member & CME Services via e-mail at *aapa@aapa.org* or call 703/836-2272, ext. 3350.

Q. Will my employer pay my AAPA dues?

A. Many employers find value with employees belonging to their professional organizations and often will pay or reimburse you for your AAPA membership. A good time to address this important issue is when you are reviewing a company's benefits during the interview process or when you are negotiating your employment contract. If you are already employed, approach your human resources department with the issue and illustrate the value you can bring to the workplace by belonging to your professional association.

Q. Are there opportunities for a new fellow member to become actively involved with the Academy?

A. Yes, there are numerous ways for you get involved from the start and assist AAPA in strengthening the unified voice of the PA profession. Here are just a few ways to participate.

- Become active in your state chapter and/or specialty organization
- Become active in an AAPA committee or council
- For more fellowship leadership opportunities, visit the PA Development Toolbox at *www.aapa.org/toolbox*.

Q. Should I join my state chapter and/or specialty organization?

A. AAPA encourages state chapter and specialty organization membership, but the decision to join is yours to make. By attending state and/or specialty chapter meetings and events, you will have numerous opportunities to network with fellow PAs and participate in efforts to support issues affecting the PA profession within your state and specialty. Being actively involved in a chapter also helps you gain leadership experience and builds management-level skills — skills you might not learn on the job or through training provided to by your employer. Please note that these memberships are exclusive of AAPA membership and require that you pay each organization's annual dues. For a complete list of state and specialty chapters, visit *https://members.aapa.org/extra/constituents/chapter-menu.cfm* and *https://members.aapa.org/extra/constituents/special-menu.cfm.*

Q. How do I update my contact information?

A. To update your contact information, go to *http://members.aapa.org* and select update your contact information. Once you have logged in, you can choose the item you wish to update. You may also e-mail your contact changes to *aapa@aapa.org.* It is suggested that you look at contact information twice a year to ensure its accuracy.

Any mailings that come from the AAPA national office will use your new address immediately. However, it can take anywhere from six to eight weeks for the change to take effect with publishers who receive mailing lists from AAPA suppliers. You don't need to send address changes to the publishers — only to AAPA. Please note that AAPA does not notify the following organizations. If you have prior affiliations with these organizations, you will need to contact them directly.

AAPA Insurance Services
222 South Prospect Avenue
Park Ridge, IL 60068
Phone: 877/356-2272, ext. 5029

National Commission on Certification of PAs
12000 Findley Road, Suite 200
Duluth, GA 30097
Phone: 678/417-8100
Fax: 678/417-8135

Q. Why can't I access the Members Only section of the AAPA Web site?

A. If your membership is not current, you can't access this area of the site. Carefully review the log-in instructions and attempt again. Your User Name is your AAPA ID number and your Password is your last name as printed on your membership card with only the first letter capitalized. If you experience problems accessing the Members Only section for more than 24 hours, contact Member & CME Services at 703/836-2272, ext. 3350.

AAPA MEMBERSHIP BENEFITS & SERVICES

PROFESSIONAL DEVELOPMENT SERVICES

AAPA's Annual Conference & Discounts
Attended by more than 8,000 PAs, PA leaders, and student PAs, this event provides numerous opportunities to network, earn CME, and get updates on the latest advances in medicine and the PA profession. Members are eligible to receive registration discounts.
www.aapa.org/annual-conf

AAPA Malpractice & Disability Insurance Service
AAPA Insurance Services offers PAs competitive rates on personal liability and malpractice insurance. AAPA Insurance Services also offers an educational resource on risk management.
www.epreceptor.com/aapa_insurance

AAPA Constituent Organization Support
AAPA offers tools and information to help strengthen constituent organizations so they may better serve their members and the PA profession. Resources available include chapter and leadership development training, strategic planning, and other support programs.
www.aapa.org/cor

AAPA Publications & On-line Store Discounts
The on-line AAPA Store offers an extensive line of products to enhance your practice capabilities at discounted member prices. Offerings include AAPA logo lab coats, scrubs and apparel, educational publications, PDAs, medical software, and diagnostic equipment.
www.aapa.org/aapastore

Medem Practice Web Site Development Service
AAPA members can build practice Web sites for themselves and physicians in their practice with Medem's Your Practice Online, an easy-to-use service to enhance the relationship between a practice and its patients.
www.aapa.org/medem.html

Networking Opportunities
Membership with AAPA offers numerous opportunities to network with leaders in the PA profession and colleagues at special events and meetings throughout the year.
www.aapa.org/aapa

PA Development Toolbox
AAPA strongly encourages all members to become actively engaged in leadership activities. This resource provides a comprehensive list of leadership opportunities, self-assessment tests, and a curriculum for enhancing a PA's professional skills.
www.aapa.org/toolbox

Public Education Materials
AAPA provides free materials for members to educate the public about the PA profession and provide physicians with information about the team practice of medicine and the working relationship between physicians and PAs.
www.aapa.org/members/pr/pr.html

PA Foundation Scholarships
The PA Foundation awards scholarships to deserving PA students across the country. Scholarships are awarded on the basis of financial need, academic achievement, extracurricular activities, and future goals as a PA.
www.aapa.org/paf/app-scholarship.html

Salary Profiles
This individualized report is created for PAs seeking personalized compensation data. The customized report compiles data that is based on a PA's practice specialty, geographic region, and the population of the labor market in which the job is located.
www.aapa.org/research/salary.html

The PA Job Link
The PA Job Link is a comprehensive resource for members seeking a range of employment services including job postings, salary profiles, and contract templates to assist PAs in negotiating an employment package.
www.aapa.org/joblink

CME AND EDUCATION SERVICES

CME Home Study Programs, Enduring Materials, & Monographs

AAPA offers home study programs available in a variety of formats, enabling PAs to earn Category I CME credit. Category I CME credit is awarded with the successful completion of a post-test. Approximately 45 hours of Category I CME can be earned through AAPA-approved home study.
www.aapa.org/cme/hs-progs.html

CME Case-based On-line Opportunities

AAPA fellow members have access to 95 case-based learning opportunities through this joint project between AAPA and MedCases. Each case completed earns up to two hours of Category I CME credit. Please note that each interactive section must be completed in order to earn CME credit.
www.aapa.org/cme

CME Post-test Processing

AAPA offers fellow members the option of submitting post-tests on-line or by mail. Nonmembers may submit post-tests by mail only, along with a $20 scoring fee for each post-test. On-line post-tests are also available (fellow members only) with the opportunity to print a certificate of completion immediately.
www.aapa.org/cme/post-test.html

Topic-specific CME Series

This series specifically assists members in meeting the requirements of their state licensing board. Approximately 11 states have topic-specific CME requirements for state licensure, and this series allows only AAPA members to document credits in the specific areas mandated by their own state licensing board.
www.aapa.org/cme/topic-spec.html

PUBLICATIONS & INFORMATIONAL SERVICES

Journal of the American Academy of Physician Assistants

JAAPA is the Academy's official peer-reviewed clinical journal for the PA profession. Its award-winning articles and insightful commentary make it a must-read monthly journal for physician assistants.
www.jaapa.com

PA Prescribing Reference

The PA Prescribing Reference is a drug reference updated and published on a monthly basis. It is intended for physicians and medical professionals who rely on accurate and up-to-date prescribing information. It offers easy access to an extensive range of current and concise drug information.
www.prescribingreference.com

AAPA News

AAPA News is the Academy's award-winning biweekly newsletter containing the latest updates on the profession and the Academy, professional practice advice, and the latest in career opportunities and information.
www.aapa.org/aapa-news

Membership Information & Resources Handbook

This handbook is a comprehensive guide to all the services offered by the Academy as well as resources for PAs in practice. Among its contents are important staff and leader contact information, AAPA structure and activities, and professional practice issues.

From Program to Practice: A Guide to the PA Profession

This publication, designed for students in their last semester of study, contains the latest information on professional issues such as third-party reimbursement, malpractice insurance, prescribing and dispensing, and state licensure.
www.aapa.org/aapastore

On-line Membership Directory

Access the membership directory on-line anytime. This tool allows you to edit your personal information, update your permissions for mailing lists, search for colleagues and former schoolmates, look up officers of constituent organizations, pay your dues, and make a donation to the AAPA Political Action Committee.
https://members.aapa.org

AAPA Web Site

The AAPA Web site is the premier source of Web-based information about the PA profession and Academy services. Find information from membership services and the Academy to state laws, reimbursement, and clinical issues. Access The PA Job Link and AAPA Store for employment services and products to enhance your practice capabilities.
www.aapa.org

GOVERNMENT AFFAIRS

Federal and State Legislative Advocacy

AAPA's Government and Professional Affairs Department speaks for the PA profession when decisions that affect PAs' ability to provide patient care are being made on the national level. You can volunteer to help by becoming involved with the Congressional Visit Program or by contributing to the election of candidates who support the PA profession through the AAPA Political Action Committee. In addition, staff works with state PA associations to improve the practice environment and make it easier for you to provide quality patient care.
www.aapa.org/gandp

Reimbursement Information & Advocacy

AAPA works diligently to assure that insurance companies and other third-party payers cover the medical and surgical services PAs provide. AAPA has conducted extensive research and made this state-by-state information on Medicare, Medicaid, and third-party coverage guidelines available to PAs.
www.aapa.org/gandp/index.html#reim

Legislative Action Center

AAPA has tools that make it easy for you to be an active and effective grassroots lobbyist by utilizing the Legislative Action Center on the AAPA Web site. You can read about current issues and communicate your views to your federal and state legislators with a few quick keystrokes.
http://members.aapa.org/vocus/index.htm

PERSONAL SERVICES

Student Loan Consolidation

In conjunction with Collegiate Risk Management, Inc., AAPA offers members the opportunity to consolidate their student loans into one low payment — as much as 58 percent lower. There is no cost to consolidate and the process does not require a credit check.
www.aapa.org/membership/serve.html

Alamo/Hertz/National Car Rental Discounts

AAPA members enjoy members-only, year-round discounted rates on car rentals with these major rental chains.
www.aapa.org/membership/serve.html

Answer Financial Insurance Products

AAPA members have access to personal insurance products from Answer Financial, including life, health care, dental, and pet insurance. Many other money-saving services are also available.
www.answercenter.com/launchpages/aapa.asp

Liberty Mutual Automobile & Homeowner's Insurance

Liberty Mutual, one of the largest auto, home, and life insurers in the world, offers AAPA members specially discounted rates on personal insurance products.
www.aapa.org/membership/serve.html

MBNA Bank Financial Services

Support AAPA and the PA profession with the only credit card officially endorsed by AAPA, the AAPA MasterCard. MBNA also offers a varied array of financial services to members.
www.mbna.com/index_main.html

Message!Check (PArtners in Medicine)

Message!Products® is the premier check printer working with nonprofits to provide personal checks, checkbook covers, address labels, and other licensed merchandise. Order your PArtners in Medicine merchandise to help increase awareness for the PA profession and support the Academy.
www.aapa.org/membership/serve.html

AAPA BENEFITS & SERVICES AVAILABLE BY MEMBERSHIP CATEGORY

	FELLOW	STUDENT
PROFESSIONAL DEVELOPMENT SERVICES		
AAPA Annual Conference Discounts	■	■
AAPA Malpractice & Disability Insurance Service	■	■
AAPA Constituent Organization Support	■	■
AAPA Publications & On-line Store Discounts	■	■
Medem Practice Web Site Development Service	■	
Networking Opportunities	■	■
PA Development Toolbox	■	■
Public Education Materials	■	■
PA Foundation Scholarships		■
Salary Profiles	■	■
The PA Job Link	■	■
CME AND EDUCATION SERVICES		
CME Home Study Programs / Enduring Materials / Monographs	■	
CME Case-based On-line Opportunities	■	
CME Post-test Processing	■	
Topic-specific CME Series	■	
PUBLICATIONS & INFORMATION SERVICES		
AAPA Web Site	■	■
Journal of the AAPA	■	■
PA Prescribing Reference	■	
Biweekly *AAPA News*	■	■
Membership Information & Resources Handbook	■	■
From Program to Practice		■
On-line Membership Directory	■	■
GOVERNMENT AFFAIRS		
Federal & State Legislative Advocacy	■	■
Reimbursement Information & Advocacy	■	■
Legislative Action Center	■	■
PERSONAL SERVICES		
Alamo / Hertz / National Rental Discounts	■	■
Answer Financial Insurance Products	■	■
Liberty Mutual Automobile & Homeowner's Insurance	■	■
MBNA Bank Financial Services	■	■
Membership Certificate	■	
Message!Check (PArtners in Medicine)	■	■
Student Loan Consolidation	■	■

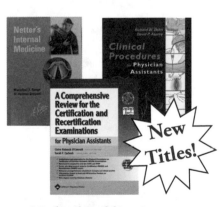
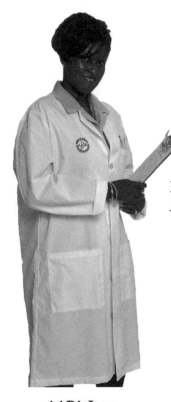
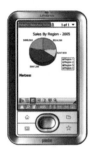
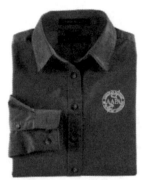
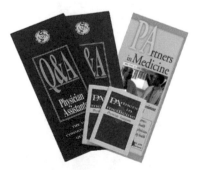

Section XII

TOOLS &
RESOURCES

DEFINITION OF "PHYSICIAN ASSISTANT"

The AAPA defines "physician assistant" as follows:

Physician assistants are health *professionals*[1] *licensed*[2] or, in the case of those employed by the federal government, credentialed, to *practice medicine with physician supervision.*[3] Physician assistants are qualified by *graduation from an accredited physician assistant educational program and/or certification by the National Commission on Certification of Physician Assistants.*[4] Within the physician/PA relationship, *physician assistants exercise autonomy in medical decision making and provide a broad range of diagnostic and therapeutic services.*[5] The clinical role of physician assistants includes *primary and specialty care in medical and surgical practice settings in rural and urban areas. Physician assistant practice is centered on patient care and may include educational, research, and administrative activities.*[6]

AAPA Policy, Adopted 1995, Amended 1996

The *Journal of the American Academy of Physician Assistants* (*JAAPA*) in January 1996 published the following explanations for the definition of "physician assistant" developed by the Professional Practice Council (PPC).

1 professionals: Recognizes the scope of PA practice, advanced knowledge required to be a PA, exercise of discretion and judgment, use of ethical standards, and orientation toward service.

2 licensed: May be of concern to PAs accustomed to the terms "certified" and "registered." Examination of accepted definitions of occupational regulation reveals, however, that PAs are subject to de facto licensure regardless of terminology employed by the state.

Experts define registration as the least restrictive form of regulation. It is a process of creating an official record or list of persons; for example, voter registration. Its main purpose is not to assure the public of qualified practitioners, but rather to perform a record-keeping function.

Under a certification system, practice of an activity or occupation is not directly restricted, but limits are placed on the use of certain occupational titles. The label "certified" publicly identifies persons who have met certain standards, but it does not prevent uncertified practitioners from engaging in the activity.

Under licensure, the most restrictive method of regulation, persons have no right to engage in a particular activity without permission to do so by the state. Such permission is generally conditional upon stringent requirements, such as certain educational qualifications and passage of an examination.

Because PAs must meet such standards and may not practice without state approval, the council believes that "licensed" is the most appropriate way to describe the control exercised by states over PA practice.

3 practice medicine with physician supervision: Consistent with AAPA policy.

4 graduation from an accredited physician assistant educational program and/or certification by the National Commission on Certification of Physician Assistants: The two major criteria for being a PA. The connector "and/or" is in accord with AAPA policy, which recognizes that informally trained, nationally certified PAs are an integral part of the profession.

5 physician assistants exercise autonomy in medical decision making and provide a broad range of diagnostic and therapeutic services: Reinforces the concept of team practice, yet emphasizes the ability of PAs to think independently when making diagnoses and clinical decisions. Also refers to the broad scope of services that PAs provide.

6 primary and specialty care in medical and surgical practice settings in rural and urban areas. Physician assistant practice is centered on patient care and may include educational, research, and administrative activities: Addresses the versatility of the PA profession, distribution of the profession in all geographic regions, and nonclinical roles that PAs may pursue.

GUIDELINES FOR ETHICAL CONDUCT

GUIDELINES FOR ETHICAL CONDUCT FOR THE PHYSICIAN ASSISTANT PROFESSION

Policy of the American Academy of Physician Assistants, adopted May 2000

INTRODUCTION

The physician assistant profession has revised its code of ethics several times since the profession began. Although the fundamental principles underlying the ethical care of patients have not changed, the societal framework in which those principles are applied has. Economic pressures of the health care system, social pressures of church and state, technological advances, and changing patient demographics continually transform the landscape in which PAs practice.

Previous codes of the profession were brief lists of tenets for PAs to live by in their professional lives. This document departs from that format by attempting to describe ways in which those tenets apply. Each situation is unique. Individual PAs must use their best judgment in a given situation while considering the preferences of the patient and the supervising physician, clinical information, ethical concepts, and legal obligations.

Four main bioethical principles broadly guided the development of these guidelines: autonomy, beneficence, nonmaleficence, and justice.

Autonomy, strictly speaking, means self-rule. Patients have the right to make autonomous decisions and choices, and physician assistants should respect these decisions and choices.

Beneficence means that PAs should act in the patient's best interest. In certain cases, respecting the patient's autonomy and acting in their best interests may be difficult to balance.

Nonmaleficence means to do no harm, to impose no unnecessary or unacceptable burden upon the patient.

Justice means that patients in similar circumstances should receive similar care. Justice also applies to norms for the fair distribution of resources, risks, and costs.

Physician assistants are expected to behave both legally and morally. They should know and understand the laws governing their practice. Likewise, they should understand the ethical responsibilities of being a health care professional. Legal requirements and ethical expectations will not always be in agreement. Generally speaking, the law describes minimum standards of acceptable behavior, and ethical principles delineate the highest moral standards of behavior.

When faced with an ethical dilemma, PAs may find the guidance they need in this document. If not, they may wish to seek guidance elsewhere — possibly from a supervising physician, a hospital ethics committee, an ethicist, trusted colleagues, or other AAPA policies. PAs should seek legal counsel when they are concerned about the potential legal consequences of their decisions.

The following sections discuss ethical conduct of PAs in their professional interactions with patients, physicians, colleagues, other health professionals, and the public. The "Statement of Values" within this document defines the fundamental values that the PA profession strives to uphold. These values provide the foundation upon which the guidelines rest. The guidelines were written with the understanding that no document can encompass all actual and potential ethical responsibilities, and PAs should not regard them as comprehensive.

Statement of Values of the Physician Assistant Profession

- Physician assistants hold as their primary responsibility the health, safety, welfare, and dignity of all human beings.
- Physician assistants uphold the tenets of patient autonomy, beneficence, nonmaleficence, and justice.
- Physician assistants recognize and promote the value of diversity.
- Physician assistants treat equally all persons who seek their care.
- Physician assistants hold in confidence the information shared in the course of practicing medicine.
- Physician assistants assess their personal capabilities and limitations, striving always to improve their medical practice.
- Physician assistants actively seek to expand their knowledge and skills, keeping abreast of advances in medicine.
- Physician assistants work with other members of the health care team to provide compassionate and effective care of patients.

- Physician assistants use their knowledge and experience to contribute to an improved community.
- Physician assistants respect their professional relationship with physicians.
- Physician assistants share and expand knowledge within the profession.

The PA and Patient

PA Role and Responsibilities

Physician assistant practice flows out of a unique relationship that involves the PA, the physician, and the patient. The individual patient–PA relationship is based on mutual respect and an agreement to work together regarding medical care. In addition, PAs practice medicine with physician supervision; therefore, the care that a PA provides is an extension of the care of the supervising physician. The patient–PA relationship is also a patient–PA–physician relationship.

The principal value of the physician assistant profession is to respect the health, safety, welfare, and dignity of all human beings. This concept is the foundation of the patient–PA relationship. Physician assistants have an ethical obligation to see that each of their patients receives appropriate care. PAs should recognize that each patient is unique and has an ethical right to self-determination. PAs should be sensitive to the beliefs and expectations of the patient, but are not expected to ignore their own personal values, scientific or ethical standards, or the law.

A PA has an ethical duty to offer each patient the full range of information on relevant options for their health care. If personal moral, religious, or ethical beliefs prevent a PA from offering the full range of treatments available or care the patient desires, the PA has an ethical duty to refer an established patient to another qualified provider. PAs are obligated to care for patients in emergency situations and to responsibly transfer established patients if they cannot care for them.

The PA and Diversity

The physician assistant should respect the culture, values, beliefs, and expectations of the patient.

Nondiscrimination

Physician assistants should not discriminate against classes or categories of patients in the delivery of needed health care. Such classes and categories include gender, color, creed, race, religion, age, ethnic or national origin, political beliefs, nature of illness, disability, socioeconomic status, or sexual orientation.

Initiation and Discontinuation of Care

In the absence of a preexisting patient-PA relationship, the physician assistant is under no ethical obligation to care for a person unless no other provider is available. A PA is morally bound to provide care in emergency situations and to arrange proper follow-up. PAs should keep in mind that contracts with health insurance plans might define a legal obligation to provide care to certain patients.

A physician assistant and supervising physician may discontinue their professional relationship with an established patient as long as proper procedures are followed. The PA and physician should provide the patient with adequate notice, offer to transfer records, and arrange for continuity of care if the patient has an ongoing medical condition. Discontinuation of the professional relationship should be undertaken only after a serious attempt has been made to clarify and understand the expectations and concerns of all involved parties.

If the patient decides to terminate the relationship, they are entitled to access appropriate information contained within their medical record.

Informed Consent

Physician assistants have a duty to protect and foster an individual patient's free and informed choices. The doctrine of informed consent means that a PA provides adequate information that is comprehendible to a competent patient or patient surrogate. At a minimum, this should include the nature of the medical condition, the objectives of the proposed treatment, treatment options, possible outcomes, and the risks involved. PAs should be committed to the concept of shared decision making, which involves assisting patients in making decisions that account for medical, situational, and personal factors. In caring for adolescents, the PA should understand all of the laws and regulations in his or her jurisdiction that are related to the ability of minors to consent to or refuse health care. Adolescents should be encouraged to involve their families in health care decision making. The PA should also understand consent laws pertaining to emancipated or mature minors. (See the section on Confidentiality.)

When the person giving consent is a patient's surrogate, a family member, or other legally authorized representative, the PA should take reasonable care to assure that the decisions made are consistent with the patient's best interests and personal preferences, if known. If the PA believes the surrogate's choices do not reflect the patient's wishes or best interests, the PA should work to resolve the conflict. This may require the use of additional resources, such as an ethics committee.

Confidentiality

Physician assistants should maintain confidentiality. By maintaining confidentiality, PAs respect patient privacy and help to prevent discrimination based on medical conditions. If patients are confident that their privacy is protected, they are more likely to seek medical care and more likely to discuss their problems candidly.

In cases of adolescent patients, family support is important but should be balanced with the patient's need for confidentiality and the PA's obligation to respect their emerging autonomy. Adolescents may not be of age to make independent decisions about their health, but providers should respect that they soon will be. To the extent they can, PAs should allow these emerging adults to participate as fully as possible in decisions about their care. It is important that PAs be familiar with and understand the laws and regulations in their jurisdictions that relate to the confidentiality rights of adolescent patients. (See the section on Informed Consent.)

Any communication about a patient conducted in a manner that violates confidentiality is unethical. Because written, electronic, and verbal information may be intercepted or overheard, the PA should always be aware of anyone who might be monitoring communication about a patient.

PAs should choose methods of storage and transmission of patient information that minimize the likelihood of data becoming available to unauthorized persons or organizations. Modern technologies such as computerized record keeping and electronic data transmission present unique challenges that can make the maintenance of patient confidentiality difficult. PAs should advocate for policies and procedures that secure the confidentiality of patient information.

The Patient and the Medical Record

Physician assistants have an obligation to keep information in the patient's medical record confidential. Information should be released only with the written permission of the patient or the patient's legally authorized representative. Specific exceptions to this general rule may exist (e.g., workers compensation, communicable disease, HIV, knife/gunshot wounds, abuse, substance abuse). It is important that a PA be familiar with and understand the laws and regulations in his or her jurisdiction that relate to the release of information. For example, stringent legal restrictions on release of genetic test results and mental health records often exist.

Both ethically and legally, a patient has certain rights to know the information contained in his or her medical record. While the chart is legally the property of the practice or the institution, the information in the chart is the property of the patient. Most states have laws that provide patients access to their medical records. The PA should know the laws and facilitate patient access to the information.

Disclosure

A physician assistant should disclose to his or her supervising physician information about errors made in the course of caring for a patient. The supervising physician and PA should disclose the error to the patient if such information is significant to the patient's interests and well being. Errors do not always constitute improper, negligent or unethical behavior, but failure to disclose them may.

Care of Family Members and Co-workers

Treating oneself, co-workers, close friends, family members, or students whom the physician assistant supervises or teaches may be unethical or create conflicts of interest. PAs should be aware that their judgment might be less than objective in cases involving friends, family members, students, and colleagues and that providing "curbside" care might sway the individual from establishing an ongoing relationship with a provider. If it becomes necessary to treat a family member or close associate, a formal patient-provider relationship should be established, and the PA should consider transferring the patient's care to another provider as soon as it is practical. If a close associate requests care, the PA may wish to assist by helping them find an appropriate provider.

There may be exceptions to this guideline, for example, when a PA runs an employee health center or works in occupational medicine. Even in those situations, PAs should be sure they do not provide informal treatment, but provide appropriate medical care in a formally established patient-provider relationship.

Genetic Testing

Evaluating the risk of disease and performing diagnostic genetic tests raise significant ethical concerns. Physician assistants should be knowledgeable about the benefits and risks of genetic tests. Testing should be undertaken only after the patient's informed consent is obtained. If PAs order or conduct the tests, they should assure that appropriate pre- and post-test counseling is provided. PAs should be sure that patients understand the potential consequences of undergoing genetic tests — from impact on patients themselves, possible implications for other family members, and potential use of the information by insurance companies or others who might have access to the information. Because of the potential for discrimination by insurers, employers, or others, PAs should be particularly aware of the need for confidentiality concerning genetic test results.

Reproductive Decision Making

Patients have a right to access the full range of reproductive health care services, including fertility treatments, contraception, sterilization, and abortion. Physician assistants have an ethical obligation to provide balanced and unbiased clinical information about reproductive health care.

When the PA's personal values conflict with providing full disclosure or providing certain services such as sterilization or abortion, the PA need not become involved in that aspect of the patient's care. By referring the patient to a qualified provider, the PA fulfills their ethical obligation to ensure the patient access to all legal options.

End of Life

Among the ethical principles that are fundamental to providing compassionate care at the end of life, the most essential is recognizing that dying is a personal experience and part of the life cycle.

Physician assistants should provide patients with the opportunity to plan for end-of-life care. Advance directives, living wills, durable power of attorney, and organ donation should be discussed during routine patient visits.

PAs should assure terminally ill patients that their dignity is a priority and that relief of physical and mental suffering is paramount. PAs should exhibit non-judgmental attitudes and should assure their terminally ill patients that they will not be abandoned. To the extent possible, patient or surrogate preferences should be honored, using the most appropriate measures consistent with their choices, including alternative and non-traditional treatments. PAs should explain palliative and hospice care and facilitate patient access to those services. End-of-life care should include assessment and management of psychological, social, and spiritual or religious needs.

While respecting patients' wishes for particular treatments when possible, PAs also must weigh their ethical responsibility, in consultation with supervising physicians, to withhold futile treatments and to help patients understand such medical decisions.

PAs should involve the physician in all near-death planning. The PA should only withdraw life support with the supervising physician's agreement and in accordance with the policies of the health care institution.

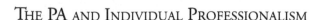

THE PA AND INDIVIDUAL PROFESSIONALISM

Conflict of Interest

Physician assistants should place service to patients before personal material gain and should avoid undue influence on their clinical judgment. Trust can be undermined by even the appearance of improper influence. Examples of excessive or undue influence on clinical judgment can take several forms. These may include financial incentives, pharmaceutical or other industry gifts, and business arrangements involving referrals. PAs should disclose any actual or potential conflict of interest to their patients.

Acceptance of gifts, trips, hospitality, or other items is discouraged. Before accepting a gift or financial arrangement, PAs might consider the guidelines of the Royal College of Physicians, "Would I be willing to have this arrangement generally known?" or of the American College of Physicians-American Society of Internal Medicine, "What would the public or my patients think of this arrangement?"

Professional Identity

Physician assistants should not misrepresent, directly or indirectly, their skills, training, professional credentials, or identity. Physician assistants should uphold the dignity of the PA profession and accept its ethical values.

Competency

Physician assistants should commit themselves to providing competent medical care and extend to each patient the full measure of their professional ability as dedicated, empathetic health care providers. PAs should also strive to maintain and increase the quality of their health care knowledge, cultural sensitivity, and cultural competence through individual study and continuing education.

Sexual Relationships

It is unethical for physician assistants to become sexually involved with patients. It also may be unethical for PAs to become sexually involved with former patients or key third parties. Key third parties are individuals who have influence over the patient. These might include spouses or partners, parents, guardians, or surrogates.

Such relationships generally are unethical because of the PA's position of authority and the inherent imbalance of knowledge, expertise, and status. Issues such as dependence, trust, transference, and inequalities of power may lead to increased vulnerability on the part of the current or former patients or key third parties.

Gender Discrimination and Sexual Harassment

It is unethical for physician assistants to engage in or condone any form of gender discrimination. Gender discrimination is defined as any behavior, action, or policy that adversely affects an individual or group of individuals due to disparate treatment, disparate impact, or the creation of a hostile or intimidating work or learning environment.

It is unethical for PAs to engage in or condone any form of sexual harassment. Sexual harassment is defined as unwelcome sexual advances, requests for sexual favors, or other verbal or physical conduct of a sexual nature when:

- Such conduct has the purpose or effect of interfering with an individual's work or academic performance or creating an intimidating, hostile or offensive work or academic environment, *or*
- Accepting or rejecting such conduct affects or may be perceived to affect professional decisions concerning an individual, *or*
- Submission to such conduct is made either explicitly or implicitly a term or condition of an individual's training or professional position.

THE PA AND OTHER PROFESSIONALS

Team Practice

Physician assistants should be committed to working collegially with other members of the health care team to assure integrated, well-managed, and effective care of patients. PAs should strive to maintain a spirit of cooperation with other health care professionals, their organizations, and the general public.

Illegal and Unethical Conduct

Physician assistants should not participate in or conceal any activity that will bring discredit or dishonor to the PA profession. They should report illegal or unethical conduct by health care professionals to the appropriate authorities.

Impairment

Physician assistants have an ethical responsibility to protect patients and the public by identifying and assisting impaired colleagues. "Impaired" means being unable to practice medicine with reasonable skill and safety because of physical or mental illness, loss of motor skills, or excessive use or abuse of drugs and alcohol.

PAs should be able to recognize impairment in physician supervisors, PAs, and other health care providers and should seek assistance from appropriate resources to encourage these individuals to obtain treatment.

PA-Physician Relationship

Supervision should include ongoing communication between the physician and the physician assistant regarding patient care. The PA should consult the supervising physician whenever it will safeguard or advance the welfare of the patient. This includes seeking assistance in situations of conflict with a patient or another health care professional.

Complementary and Alternative Medicine

A patient's request for alternative therapy may create conflict between the physician assistant and the patient. Though physician assistants are under no obligation to provide an alternative therapy, they do have a responsibility to be sensitive to the patient's needs and beliefs and to help the patient understand their medical condition. The PA should gain an understanding of the alternative therapy being considered or being used, the expected outcome, and whether the treatment would clearly be harmful to the patient. If the treatment would harm the patient, the PA should work diligently to dissuade the patient from using it and advise other treatment.

The PA and the Health Care System

Workplace Actions

Physician assistants may face difficult personal decisions to withhold medical services when workplace actions (e.g., strikes, sick-outs, slowdowns) occur. The potential harm to patients should be carefully weighed against the potential improvements to working conditions and, ultimately, patient care that could result. In general, PAs should individually and collectively work to find alternatives to such actions in addressing workplace concerns.

Managed Care

The focus of managed care organizations on cost containment and resource allocation can present particular ethical challenges to clinicians. When practicing in managed care systems, physician assistants should always act in the best interests of their patients and as an advocate when necessary. PAs should actively resist managed care policies that restrict free exchange of medical information. For example, a PA should not withhold information about treatment options simply because the option is not covered by a particular managed care organization.

PAs should inform patients of financial incentives to limit care, use resources in a fair and efficient way, and avoid arrangements or financial incentives that conflict with the patient's best interests.

PAs as Educators

All physician assistants have a responsibility to share knowledge and information with patients, other health professionals, students, and the public. The ethical duty to teach includes effective communication with patients so that they will have the information necessary to participate in their health care and wellness.

PAs and Research

The most important ethical principle in research is honesty. This includes assuring subjects' informed consent, following treatment protocols, and accurately reporting findings. Fraud and dishonesty in research should be reported so that the appropriate authorities can take action.

Physician assistants involved in research must be aware of potential conflicts of interest. The patient's welfare takes precedence over the desired research outcome. Any conflict of interest should be disclosed.

In scientific writing, PAs should report information honestly and accurately. Sources of funding for the research must be included in the published reports.

Plagiarism is unethical. Incorporating the words of others, either verbatim or by paraphrasing, without appropriate attribution is unethical and may have legal consequences. When submitting a document for publication, any previous publication of any portion of the document must be fully disclosed.

PAs as Expert Witnesses

The physician assistant expert witness should testify to what he or she believes to be the truth. The PA's review of medical facts should be thorough, fair, and impartial.

The PA expert witness should be fairly compensated for time spent preparing, appearing, and testifying. The PA should not accept a contingency fee based on the outcome of a case in which testimony is given or derive personal, financial, or professional favor in addition to compensation.

THE PA AND SOCIETY

Lawfulness

Physician assistants have the dual duty to respect the law and to work for positive change to laws that will enhance the health and well being of the community.

Executions

Physician assistants, as health care professionals, should not participate in executions because to do so would violate the ethical principle of beneficence.

Access to Care/Resource Allocation

Physician assistants have a responsibility to use health care resources in an appropriate and efficient manner so that all patients have access to needed health care. Resource allocation should be based on societal needs and policies, not the circumstances of an individual patient–PA encounter. PAs participating in policy decisions about resource allocation should consider medical need, cost-effectiveness, efficacy, and equitable distribution of benefits and burdens in society.

Community Well Being

Physician assistants should work for the health, well being, and the best interest of both the patient and the community. Sometimes there is a dynamic moral tension between the well being of the community in general and the individual patient. Conflict between an individual patient's best interest and the common good is not always easily resolved. In general, PAs should be committed to upholding and enhancing community values, be aware of the needs of the community, and use the knowledge and experience acquired as professionals to contribute to an improved community.

CONCLUSION

The American Academy of Physician Assistants recognizes its responsibility to aid the PA profession as it strives to provide high quality, accessible health care. Physician assistants wrote these guidelines for themselves and other physician assistants. The ultimate goal is to honor patients and earn their trust while providing the best and most appropriate care possible. At the same time, PAs must understand their personal values and beliefs and recognize the ways in which those values and beliefs can impact the care they provide.

STATE REGULATORY AUTHORITIES

PHYSICIAN ASSISTANT STATE AND TERRITORIAL REGULATORY AUTHORITIES

ALABAMA, BOARD OF
MEDICAL EXAMINERS
PO Box 946
Montgomery, AL 36101-0946
334/242-4116
www.albme.org

ALASKA, MEDICAL LICENSING BOARD
Division of Occupational Licensing
550 West 7th Avenue, Suite 1500
Anchorage, AK 99501
907/269-8163
www.dced.state.ak.us/occ/pmed.htm

ARIZONA, REGULATORY BOARD
OF PHYSICIAN ASSISTANTS
9545 E Doubletree Ranch Road
Scottsdale, AZ 85258
480/551-2700
www.azpaboard.org

ARKANSAS, STATE MEDICAL BOARD
2100 Riverfront Drive, Suite 200
Little Rock, AR 72202-1793
501/296-1802
www.armedicalboard.org

CALIFORNIA, PHYSICIAN
ASSISTANT COMMITTEE
1424 Howe Avenue, #35
Sacramento, CA 95825
916/561-8780
www.physicianassistant.ca.gov

COLORADO, BOARD OF
MEDICAL EXAMINERS
1560 Broadway Street, Suite 1300
Denver, CO 80202
303/894-7690
www.dora.state.co.us/medical

CONNECTICUT, DIVISION OF
MEDICAL QUALITY ASSURANCE
Department of Public Health –
PA Licensing
410 Capitol Avenue MS #12APP
PO Box 340308
Hartford, CT 06134-0308
860/509-8000
www.ct-clic.com/detail.asp?code=1761

DELAWARE, BOARD OF
MEDICAL PRACTICE
Cannon Bldg, Suite 203
861 Silver Lake Boulevard
Dover, DE 19904-2467
302/744-4500
http://dpr.delaware.gov/boards/medi-
calpractice/index.shtml

DISTRICT OF COLUMBIA,
BOARD OF MEDICINE
717 14th St NW, Suite 600
Washington, DC 20005
202/724-4900
www.dchealth.dc.gov

FLORIDA, BOARD OF
MEDICAL EXAMINERS
4052 Bald Cypress Way, Bin # C03
Tallahassee, FL 32399-3256
850/488-0595
www.doh.state.fl.us/mqa/PhysAsst/

FLORIDA, BOARD OF OSTEOPATHIC
MEDICAL EXAMINERS
4052 Bald Cypress Way, Bin # C06
Tallahassee, FL 32399-3256
850/245-4161
www.doh.state.fl.us/mqa/osteopath

GEORGIA, COMPOSITE STATE
BOARD OF MEDICAL EXAMINERS
2 Peachtree Street NW, 36th Floor
Atlanta, GA 30303-3465
404/656-3913
www.ganet.org/meb/oa_physasst.html

GUAM, BOARD OF
MEDICAL EXAMINERS
Health Professionals Licensing Office
651 Legacy Square Commercial Complex
South Route 10, Suite 9
Margilao, GU, 96913
011/671/735-7406

HAWAII, BOARD OF
MEDICAL EXAMINERS
Dept. of Commerce & Consumer
Affairs, Division of Prof. Licensing
PO Box 3469
Honolulu, HI 96801
808/586-3000
www.state.hi.us/dcca/areas/pvl/boards/
medical

IDAHO, BOARD OF MEDICINE
PO Box 83720
Boise, ID 83720-0058
208/327-7000
www.bom.state.id.us

ILLINOIS, DIVISION OF
PROFESSIONAL REGULATION
320 West Washington Street
Springfield, IL 62786
217/785-0800
www.idfpr.com/dpr/WHO/adjmed.asp

Most PA regulatory agencies can be accessed through a Web link at
www.aapa.org/gandp/statereg.html.

INDIANA, Health
Professions Bureau
Attn: PA Committee
Medical Licensing Board
402 West Washington Street
Suite W066
Indianapolis, IN 46204
317/234-2060
www.in.gov/pla/bandc/pac

IOWA, Board of Physician
Assistant Examiners
Professional Licensing Division
Lucas State Office Building
321 East 12th Street, Capitol Complex
Des Moines, IA 50319-0075
515/281-4401
*www.idph.state.ia.us/licensure/board_
home.asp?board=pa*

KANSAS, Board of Healing Arts
235 SW Topeka Boulevard
Topeka, KS 66603-3068
785/296-7413
www.ksbha.org

KENTUCKY, Board of
Medical Licensure
310 Whittington Pkway, Suite 1B
Louisville, KY 40222
502/429-7150
*www.state.ky.us/agencies/kbml/
physicianasst.html*

LOUISIANA, Board of
Medical Examiners
PO Box 30250
New Orleans, LA 70190-0250
504/568-6820
www.lsbme.louisiana.gov

MAINE, Board of Licensure
in Medicine
137 State House Station
161 Capitol Street
Augusta, ME 04333-0137
207/287-3601
www.docboard.org/me/me_home.htm

MAINE, Board of
Osteopathic Examiners
142 State House Station
161 Capitol Street
Augusta, ME 04333
207/287-2480
www.maine.gov/osteo

MARYLAND, Board of Physicians
4201 Patterson Avenue
Baltimore, MD 21215
410/764-4777 or 800/492-6836
www.mbp.state.md.us/

MASSACHUSETTS, Board of
Physician Assistant Registration
Division of Registration
239 Causeway Street, Suite 200
Boston, MA 02114
617/973-0806
www.mass.gov/dpl/boards/ap/index.htm

MICHIGAN, Physician
Assistant Task Force
Bureau of Health Professions
PO Box 30670
Lansing, MI 48909
517/335-0918
www.michigan.gov/mdch

MINNESOTA, Board of
Medical Practice
2829 University Avenue SE, Suite 500
Minneapolis, MN 55414-3246
612/617-2130
www.bmp.state.mn.us

MISSISSIPPI, Board of
Medical Licensure
1867 Crane Ridge Drive, Suite 200B
Jackson, MS 39216
601/987-3079
www.msbml.state.ms.us

MISSOURI, Board of
Registration for the Healing Arts
State Advisory Commission
for Physician Assistants
PO Box 4
Jefferson City, MO 65102
573/751-0098
http://pr.mo.gov/physicianassistants.asp

MONTANA, Board of
Medical Examiners
PO Box 200513
Helena, MT 59620-0513
406/841-2300
*http://www.mt.gov/dli/bsd/license/
bsd_boards/med_board/licenses/med/
lic_pac.asp*

NEBRASKA, Health Department
Board of Examiners in Medicine
and Surgery
PO Box 94986
Lincoln, NE 68509-4986
402/471-2115
www.hhs.state.ne.us/crl/crlindex.htm

NEVADA, Board of
Medical Examiners
PO Box 7238
Reno, NV 89510
775/688-2559 or 888/890-8210
www.state.nv.us/medical

NEVADA, State Board of
Osteopathic Medicine
2860 E. Flamingo Road, Suite D
Las Vegas, NV 89121-5208
702/732-2147
www.osteo.state.nv.us

NEW HAMPSHIRE,
Board of Medicine
2 Industrial Park Drive, Suite 8
Concord, NH 03301-8520
603/271-1203
www.nh.gov/medicine/pai.html

NEW JERSEY, PHYSICIAN
ASSISTANT ADVISORY COMMITTEE
PO Box 45035
Newark, NJ 07101
973/504-6580
www.state.nj.us/lps/ca/medical/pa.htm

NEW JERSEY, BOARD OF
MEDICAL EXAMINERS
PO Box 183
Trenton, NJ 08625-0183
609/826-7100
www.state.nj.us/lps/ca/medical/bme.htm

NEW MEXICO, MEDICAL BOARD
2055 South Pacheco Street
Building 400
Santa Fe, NM 87505
505/476-7220 or 800/945-5845
http://nmmb.state.nm.us

NEW MEXICO, BOARD OF
OSTEOPATHIC MEDICAL EXAMINERS
2550 Cerrillos Road
Santa Fe, NM 87505
505/476-7120
http://www.rld.state.nm.us/b&c/osteo/
index.htm

NEW YORK, STATE BOARD
FOR MEDICINE
Office of the Professions
State Education Building, 2nd Floor
Albany, NY 12234
518/474-3817
www.op.nysed.gov/rpa.htm

NORTH CAROLINA,
MEDICAL BOARD
PO Box 20007
Raleigh, NC 27619-0007
919/326-1100
www.ncmedboard.org

NORTH DAKOTA,
BOARD OF MEDICAL EXAMINERS
418 East Broadway Avenue, Suite 12
Bismarck, ND 58501
701/328-6500
www.ndbomex.com

NORTHERN MARIANAS
ISLANDS, MEDICAL PROFESSIONAL
LICENSING BOARD
PO Box 501458
CK, Saipan MP 96950
670/664-4811
www.cnmi-guide.com

OHIO, STATE MEDICAL BOARD
77 South High Street, 17th Floor
Columbus, OH 43215-6127
614/466-3934
http://med.ohio.gov/PAsubwebindex.htm

OKLAHOMA, BOARD OF MEDICAL
LICENSURE AND SUPERVISION
PO Box 18256
Oklahoma City, OK 73154-0256
405/848-6841
www.osbmls.state.ok.us

OREGON, BOARD OF
MEDICAL EXAMINERS
1500 SW First Avenue, Suite 620
Portland, OR 97201
503/229-5770 or 877/254-6263
http://egov.oregon.gov/BME

PENNSYLVANIA,
BOARD OF MEDICINE
PO Box 2649
Harrisburg, PA 17105-2649
717/783-1400
www.dos.state.pa.us/bpoa/medbd/
mainpage.htm

PENNSYLVANIA, BOARD OF
OSTEOPATHIC MEDICINE
PO Box 2649
Harrisburg, PA 17105-2649
717/783-4858
www.dos.state.pa.us/bpoa/ostbd/
mainpage.htm

RHODE ISLAND, BOARD OF
PHYSICIAN ASSISTANTS
Division of Health Services Regulation
Health Professionals
3 Capitol Hill, Room 104
Providence, RI 02908
401/222-2827
www.healthri.org/hsr/professions/
phys_assist.php

SOUTH CAROLINA,
BOARD OF MEDICAL EXAMINERS
PO Box 11289
Columbia, SC 29211-1289
803/896-4500
www.llr.state.sc.us/POL/Medical

SOUTH DAKOTA, BOARD OF
MEDICAL AND OSTEOPATHIC EXAMINERS
1323 South Minnesota Avenue
Sioux Falls, SD 57105
605/336-1965
www.state.sd.us/doh/medical/index.htm

TENNESSEE, PHYSICIAN
ASSISTANT COMMITTEE, DEPARTMENT
OF HEALTH-RELATED BOARDS
Cordell Hull Building
425 5th Avenue North
Nashville, TN 37247-1010
615/532-3202 or 800/778-4123
http://www2.state.tn.us/health/boards/
PA/index.htm

TEXAS, PHYSICIAN ASSISTANT BOARD
c/o Texas Medical Board
PO Box 2018
Austin, TX 78768-2018
512/305-7022
www.tsbme.state.tx.us

UTAH, PHYSICIAN ASSISTANT
LICENSING BOARD
Division of Occupational and
Prof. Licensing
PO Box 146741
Salt Lake City, UT 84114-6741
801/530-6628
www.dopl.utah.gov

VERMONT, BOARD OF
MEDICAL PRACTICE
PO Box 70
Burlington, VT 05402-0070
802/657-4220
http://www.healthyvermonters.info/
bmp/bmp.shtml

VIRGIN ISLANDS, BOARD
OF MEDICAL EXAMINERS
Department of Health
48 Sugar Estate
St. Thomas, VI 00802
340/774-0117

VIRGINIA, BOARD OF MEDICINE
6603 West Broad Street, 5th Floor
Richmond, VA 23230-1712
804/662-9908
www.dhp.state.va.us/medicine/
default.htm

WASHINGTON, STATE
DEPARTMENT OF HEALTH
Health Professions Quality Assurance
PO Box 47865
Olympia, WA 98504-7865
360/236-4700
https://fortress.wa.gov/doh/hpqa1/
HPS5/Medical/default.htm

WASHINGTON, BOARD OF OSTEO-
PATHIC MEDICINE & SURGERY
Health Professions Quality Assurance
PO Box 47865
Olympia, WA 98504-7865
360/236-4700
https://fortress.wa.gov/doh/hpqa1/
hps7/osteopath/default.htm

WEST VIRGINIA, BOARD
OF MEDICINE
101 Dee Drive, Suite 103
Charleston, WV 25311
304/558-2921
www.wvdhhr.org/wvbom

WEST VIRGINIA,
BOARD OF OSTEOPATHY
334 Penco Road
Weirton, WV 26062
304/723-4638
www.wvbdosteo.org

WISCONSIN, MEDICAL
EXAMINING BOARD
PO Box 8935
Madison, WI 53708-8935
608/266-2112
http://drl.wi.gov/prof/phya/def.htm

WYOMING, BOARD OF MEDICINE
211 W. 19th Street, 2nd Floor
Colony Building
Cheyenne, WY 82002
307/778-7053
http://wyomedboard.state.wy.us

AAPA Issue Briefs

Issue Briefs on the following topics are available on AAPA's Web site at *www.aapa.org/gandp/issuebrief* or from AAPA's Government and Professional Affairs Department. Call 703/836-2272, ext. 3207.

PROFESSIONAL ISSUES
- The Physician-PA Team
- Physician Assistant Scope of Practice
- Physician Assistants and Protocols
- Medical Unions and Physician Assistants
- Hiring a PA: The Benefits for Physicians and Practices
- Physician Assistants as Shareholders in Professional Corporations
- Independent Practice Associations (IPAs): A Primer for Physician Assistants

EDUCATION
- Physician Assistant Education: Preparation for Excellence
- PA Prescribing: Education and Delegation
- Physician Assistants as Prescribers of Controlled Medications
- Physician Assistants and Anesthesiologist Assistants: The Distinctions
- Physician Assistants and Orthopedic Physician Assistants: The Distinctions
- Physician Assistants in Hospital Practice: Credentialing and Privileging
- Physician Assistants in Hospital Practice: Credentialing and Privileging
- Denial of Hospital Privileges: Antitrust Implications
- Physician Assistants as Members of the Medical Staff

SPECIALTY PRACTICE
- Introducing Surgical Physician Assistants
- Physician Assistants in Surgery
- Physician Assistants in Allergy and Immunology Medicine
- Physician Assistants and Cardiology
- Physician Assistants in Dermatology
- Physician Assistants in Gastroenterology and Hepatology
- Physician Assistants in Emergency Medicine
- Physician Assistants in Nephrology
- Physician Assistants in Oncology
- Physician Assistants in Orthopedic Surgery
- Physician Assistants in Otolaryngology
- Occupational Medicine PAs: Promoting Employee Health
- Physician Assistants and Radiology
- Physician Assistants and Radiology Practitioner Assistants: The Distinctions
- Physician Assistants and Women's Health
- Physician Assistants in Pediatrics
- Meeting Rural America's Needs: PA Presence Remains Strong

REIMBURSEMENT ISSUES
- Third Party Reimbursement for Physician Assistants
- Medicare Provisions Affecting Physician Assistants in the Balanced Budget Act of 1997
- Medicare's Final Rule on Billing Requirements for Teaching Physicians
- Coverage and Payment for Services: Antitrust Issues
- Antitrust Implications of Negotiating with Third Party Payers

STATE GOVERNMENT ISSUES
- Ratio of Physician Assistants to Supervising Physicians
- The Role of Physician Assistants in Evaluating and Certifying Health Status
- Standardization of Regulatory Terms: Licensure for Physician Assistants
- State Children's Health Insurance Program
- The Role of Chart Co-signature in Physician Supervision of Physician Assistants
- Physician Assistants and Medical Response to Disasters and Emergencies: Amending State Laws

OTHER AAPA RESOURCES
The following publications are available from the AAPA store. Order on-line at *www.aapa.org/aapastore*.
- *Hiring a Physician Assistant*
- *Physician Assistants and Hospital Practice*
- *Physician Assistant Third Party Coverage*
- *Physician Assistants: State Laws and Regulations*
- *Annotated Bibliography of the Physician Assistant Profession*
- *Addendum to the Annotated Bibliography, 1993-1999*

Available on the Web at *www.aapa.org/gandp/propractopref. html* or from the AAPA Government and Professional Affairs Department:
- Professional Practice Topics and References, a bibliography of resources prepared by the AAPA Professional Practice Council

Available from the AAPA Data Systems and Analysis Department:
- Information Updates, short, informative articles based on information from the AAPA Annual PA Census Survey and the AAPA Annual Conference Survey, including information on salary, fringe benefits, number of PAs in clinical practice, and types of disorders PAs see.

CENSUS INFORMATION: PA INCOMES & FRINGE BENEFITS

INCOME REPORTED BY PAs WHO GRADUATED IN 2004

OVERVIEW

Results of the 2005 AAPA Physician Assistant Census Survey indicate the mean total income for clinically practicing PAs who work full-time (32 or more hours a week) for their primary employer and who graduated in 2004 is $68,116 (standard deviation of $13,077); the median is $66,591. A summary of the personal and practice characteristics of the new graduate respondents and a set of tables showing summary measures of their incomes in total, by region of the country and by area of general specialty, are presented below.

PERSONAL CHARACTERISTICS

Sex: Seventy-four percent of these new graduate respondents were female.

Race/Ethnicity: Eighty-five percent reported that they were white (not Hispanic), 6 percent reported that they were Asian, 5 percent reported that they were Hispanic/Latino, and 5 percent reported that they were black (not Hispanic).

Age: The mean age of these respondents was 31 years; the median age was 28. The youngest 10 percent were 25 years or younger; the oldest 10 percent were 40 years or older.

PRACTICE CHARACTERISTICS

Employer type: A single or multispecialty physician group practice employed 43 percent of these respondents. Twenty-three percent of the respondents were employed by hospitals, and 17 percent were employed by a solo physician practice. Work setting: The predominant work setting for the respondents was a solo or group practice office (47%). More than one-third of the respondents (37%) worked in a hospital, and another seven percent worked in some type of Federally Qualified Health Center or community health facility.

Hours worked: The mean hours worked per week by the respondents who reported full-time employment was 45.4; the median was 45 hours per week.

Call: Forty percent of these respondents reported taking call. The mean hours on call per month for those who reported taking call was 90; the median was 60.

INCOME

Table 1. Summary Measures of Total Annual Income from Primary Employer for Respondents Who Graduated in 2004 and Work at Least 32 Hours per Week at their Primary Clinical Job*

	Total
Respondents	1,866
Mean	$ 68,116
Standard Deviation	$ 13,077
10th percentile	$ 54,716
25th percentile	$ 60,571
Median	$ 66,591
75th percentile	$ 73,891
90th percentile	$ 83,555

*Excludes self-employed PAs and part-time PAs.
©2005 AAPA 10/6/2005

Table 2. Summary Measures of Total Annual Income from Primary Clinical Job for Respondents Who Graduated in 2004, by Region *

	Northeast	Southeast	North Central	South Central	West	Total
Respondents	412	419	404	254	321	1866
Mean	$65,964	$68,234	$67,545	$69,647	$70,163	$68,116
Standard Deviation	$11,759	$13,697	$11,799	$14,529	$13,667	$13,077
10th percentile	$52,980	$54,810	$55,360	$57,258	$56,003	$54,716
25th percentile	$57,812	$60,340	$60,599	$61,891	$61,833	$60,571
Median	$64,881	$66,266	$66,200	$67,641	$68,303	$66,591
75th percentile	$71,888	$74,276	$72,647	$74,414	$77,458	$73,891
90th percentile	$80,410	$84,082	$80,698	$84,337	$90,092	$83,555

Excludes self-employed PAs and part-time PAs. ©2005 AAPA 10/6/2005

Table 3. Summary Measures of Total Annual Income from Primary Employer at Primary Clinical Job for Respondents Who Graduated in 2004, by Area of General Specialty*

	Respondents	Mean	Standard Deviation	10th Percentile	25th Percentile	Median	75th Percentile	90th Percentile
Family/general medicine	454	$63,521	$11,554	$50,741	$56,963	$62,935	$69,377	$74,904
General internal medicine	118	$66,928	$11,648	$55,675	$59,717	$65,382	$70,848	$78,803
Emergency medicine	142	$76,553	$14,001	$61,029	$66,241	$74,044	$83,699	$95,630
General pediatrics	49	$64,522	$11,685	$50,570	$56,698	$63,080	$72,088	$76,854
General surgery	83	$67,543	$11,437	$57,003	$62,097	$67,583	$73,463	$78,349
Internal medicine subspecialties	256	$67,342	$10,967	$55,515	$60,918	$66,329	$73,207	$80,403
Pediatric subspecialties	39	$66,850	$10,769	$53,424	$61,082	$66,642	$71,845	$77,695
Surgical subspecialties	462	$72,125	$13,296	$58,400	$63,982	$70,008	$78,405	$87,492
Obstetrics and gynecology	48	$62,479	$14,281	$44,712	$55,128	$63,535	$68,810	$80,218
Other	210	$67,552	$14,052	$52,611	$59,315	$65,788	$73,711	$82,066
Total	1866	$68,116	$13,077	$54,716	$60,571	$66,591	$73,891	$83,555

Excludes self-employed PAs and part-time PAs. ©2005 AAPA 10/6/2005

AAPA Physician Assistant Census Results: Fringe Benefits

Each year, AAPA conducts a census survey of physician assistants to collect information on the profession. The following information, taken from the 2004 and 2005 AAPA Physician Assistant Census Surveys, summarizes some of the employment benefits received by PAs who work 32 or more hours per week for their primary employer and who are not self-employed.

ANNUAL PAID LEAVE

The majority of respondents to the 2005 AAPA Census (81%) reported that they accrue paid leave for distinct categories (e.g., vacation, sick, etc.); 11 percent receive a lump sum of paid leave; and 8 percent reported that they do not receive paid leave from their primary employer. Most of those who receive distinct categories of paid leave are offered paid leave for vacation (99%), illness (83%), and CME (85%). The mean number of days offered per year for these types of leave are 17, 10, and 6, respectively. (See Table 1.)

Table 1. Annual Days of Paid Vacation, Sick, and CME Leave Offered to PAs by Primary Employer

Description	Mean	Median	Standard Deviation
Annual Days of Paid Vacation Leave (n= 11,504)	17	15	6.6
Annual Days of Paid Sick Leave (n= 7,166)	10	9	7.6
Annual Days of Paid CME Leave (n= 8,506)	6	5	2.3

FUNDING FOR CONTINUING MEDICAL EDUCATION

Data regarding funding for continuing medical education (CME) were not collected in the 2005 AAPA Physician Assistant Census Survey. According to the 2004 AAPA Physician Assistant Census Survey, the vast majority (88%) of PAs received CME funding from their primary employer. The mean amount of CME funds available in 2004 for PAs who received CME funds from their primary employer was $1,559 (standard deviation=$791, median=$1,500).

OTHER FRINGE BENEFITS

Analysis of data from the 2004 AAPA Physician Assistant Census Survey indicates that professional liability insurance is the most commonly reimbursed fringe benefit for PAs and it is almost universally reimbursed at 95-100 percent. (See Table 2.)

Further analysis of these data reveals large differences between the benefit packages of PAs who receive an hourly wage compared to PAs who are salaried. Disproportionately more PAs who receive salaries than PAs who receive an hourly wage are reimbursed 95-100 percent of the cost of state license fees, DEA registration fees, NCCPA fees, AAPA dues, state PA chapter dues, AAPA annual conference fees, and credentialing fees. (See Tables 3 and 4.)

Table 2. Percentage of PAs Receiving Specified Fringe Benefits

Description	BENEFIT REIMBURSED BY EMPLOYER			
	95-100% by Employer	50-94% by Employer	1-49% by Employer	Benefit Not Reimbursed
Professional Liability Insurance (n=13,415)	97%	1%	0%	2%
Individual Health Insurance (n=12,514)	50%	35%	6%	8%
Family Health Insurance (n=9,593)	27%	35%	10%	28%
Dental Insurance (n=11,723)	32%	31%	9%	29%
Disability Insurance (n=11,285)	45%	17%	7%	31%
Term Life Insurance (n=10,719)	41%	14%	9%	36%
Pension/Retirement Fund (n=11,858)	25%	21%	35%	19%
State License Fees (n=12,824)	71%	1%	1%	27%
DEA Registration Fees (n=10,321)	75%	1%	1%	24%
NCCPA Fees (n=12,719)	63%	1%	1%	35%
AAPA Dues (n=12,701)	63%	1%	1%	35%
State PA Chapter Dues (n=11,802)	56%	1%	1%	42%
AAPA Annual Conference Fees (n=11,162)	58%	8%	4%	30%
Credentialing Fees (n=11,953)	73%	2%	1%	23%

Table 3. Percentage of Salaried PAs Receiving Specified Fringe Benefits

Description	BENEFIT REIMBURSED BY EMPLOYER			
	95-100% by Employer	50-94% by Employer	1-49% by Employer	Benefit Not Reimbursed
Professional Liability Insurance (n=10,827)	98%	1%	0%	1%
Individual Health Insurance (n=10,160)	52%	35%	6%	7%
Family Health Insurance (n=7,690)	27%	36%	10%	27%
Dental Insurance (n=9,481)	32%	31%	9%	28%
Disability Insurance (n=9,122)	46%	17%	7%	30%
Term Life Insurance (n=8,694)	43%	14%	8%	34%
Pension/Retirement Fund (n=9,601)	26%	21%	36%	17%
State License Fees (n=10,454)	75%	1%	1%	23%
DEA Registration Fees (n=8,328)	78%	1%	0%	20%
NCCPA Fees (n=10,369)	67%	1%	1%	31%
AAPA Dues (n=10,367)	67%	1%	1%	31%
State PA Chapter Dues (n=9,601)	60%	2%	1%	38%
AAPA Annual Conference Fees (n=9,052)	62%	8%	4%	27%
Credentialing Fees (n=9,735)	76%	2%	1%	20%

Table 4. Percentage of Hourly PAs Receiving Specified Fringe Benefits

Description	BENEFIT REIMBURSED BY EMPLOYER			
	95-100% by Employer	50-94% by Employer	1-49% by Employer	Benefit Not Reimbursed
Professional Liability Insurance (n=2,263)	97%	1%	0%	2%
Individual Health Insurance (n=2,043)	44%	34%	7%	15%
Family Health Insurance (n=1,647)	25%	32%	10%	33%
Dental Insurance (n=1,971)	28%	31%	9%	32%
Disability Insurance (n=1,903)	38%	19%	9%	34%
Term Life Insurance (n=1,783)	36%	14%	10%	41%
Pension/Retirement Fund (n=1,983)	22%	18%	34%	25%
State License Fees (n=2,074)	54%	2%	1%	44%
DEA Registration Fees (n=1,736)	59%	1%	1%	39%
NCCPA Fees (n=2,046)	46%	1%	1%	52%
AAPA Dues (n=2,035)	45%	1%	1%	53%
State PA Chapter Dues (n=1,914)	38%	1%	1%	60%
AAPA Annual Conference Fees (n=1,842)	40%	8%	5%	47%
Credentialing Fees (n=1,927)	60%	3%	2%	36%

AAPA SALARY PROFILE

WHAT IS A SALARY PROFILE?

A salary profile is an information tool used by PAs and employers of PAs to answer the question: "How much have PAs, in positions with certain characteristics, earned?" Salary profiles are descriptive and not prescriptive. AAPA provides them for informational purposes only and disclaims any attempt to directly or indirectly use the data to establish compensation schedules.

WHAT IS THE SOURCE OF THE DATA USED TO PRODUCE A SALARY PROFILE?

AAPA's Annual Physician Assistant Census is the source of the data used to prepare salary profiles; it is the most current and comprehensive information about PA compensation available anywhere.

WHAT CHARACTERISTICS DOES A SALARY PROFILE TAKE INTO ACCOUNT?

The position to be studied needs to be identified in terms of the specialty of practice, the geographic location of the work site, and the population of the labor market in which the job is located. Once this is established, the analyst extracts data for all PAs in the census database that meet the defined parameters.

WHAT IF THERE AREN'T ENOUGH PAs WHO WORK IN JOBS LIKE THE ONE SPECIFIED?

If there are too few PAs matching the parameters defined, the analyst expands the parameters until the sample is sufficiently large. Normally, this means including one or two neighboring states or expanding the range of populations to be accepted. Occasionally, it means using the entire United States. When this occurs, the data are still meaningful, since the labor market for such a PA position is indeed national in scope.

WHAT STATISTICS ARE REPORTED IN A SALARY PROFILE?

The following summary measures are presented for total income from primary PA job for subgroups of PAs defined by years of experience:

- Mean: the simple average of all reported incomes.
- Standard error of the mean: a measure of variation, it is used to calculate 95 percent confidence intervals by adding and subtracting two standard errors to and from the mean.
- 10th, 25th, 50th, 75th, and 90th percentiles: measures depicting the distribution of incomes in the sample. An income at the 10th percentile is greater than the income reported by 10 percent of the respondents; the median or 50th percentile represents the income that is greater than that reported by half of the respondents; etc.

WHO CAN ORDER A SALARY PROFILE?

Only AAPA members can order salary profiles. The fee for fellow and student members is $35; the fee for other members is $150.

HOW CAN A SALARY PROFILE BE ORDERED?

Orders can be placed anytime throughout the year by calling 703/836-2272, ext. 3807 or 3128.

NOTES

NOTES